A Revolution in Health through Nutritional Biochemistry

A Revolution in Health through Nutritional Biochemistry

John Neustadt, ND
Steve Pieczenik, MD, PhD

iUniverse, Inc.
New York Lincoln Shanghai

A Revolution in Health through Nutritional Biochemistry

iUniverse books may be ordered through booksellers or by contacting:

iUniverse
2021 Pine Lake Road, Suite 100
Lincoln, NE 68512
www.iuniverse.com
1-800-Authors (1-800-288-4677)

Because of the dynamic nature of the Internet, any Web addresses or links contained in this book may have changed since publication and may no longer be valid.

You should not undertake any diet recommended in this book before consulting your personal physician. Neither the author nor the publisher shall be responsible or liable for any loss or damage allegedly arising as a consequence of your use or application of any information or suggestions contained in this book.

ISBN: 978-0-595-45340-5 (pbk)
ISBN: 978-0-595-89652-3 (ebk)

Printed in the United States of America

Dr. Neustadt would like to dedicate this book to his wife, Romi. Without her patient support over the past six years of research that went into writing this book and building a clinical practice, this book would not have been possible. He also dedicates this book to his son, Nate, who inspires Dr. Neustadt to continually work harder to help create a better world and, more specifically, a better health care system for his son and the generations to come. Additionally, Dr. Neustadt would like thank Dr. Pieczenik for his guidance, mentorship, and inspiration. Without Dr. Pieczenik, this book would never have been written.

Dr. Pieczenik wishes to dedicate this book to his lodestars, Birdie, Stephanie, and Sharon, who had to tolerate living with their father in Bozeman, Montana. He also dedicates this work to all his patients whom he had treated and who had inspired him to look into alternative ways to improve their health and increase his knowledge of the true workings of both the mind and body.

Contents

Acknowledgments

The authors would like to acknowledge the pioneering work of Metametrix Clinical Laboratory. The testing services pioneered by its founder, Alexander Bralley, PhD, over the past twenty years have provided clinicians the ability to evaluate the underlying biochemical causes of disease as never before. NBI Testing and Consulting Corporation and Drs. Pieczenik and Neustadt are proud of their unique relationship with the laboratory. Based on Dr. Neustadt's research into the biochemical bases of health and disease, Metametrix hired Dr. Neustadt to edit and peer-review their textbook, *Laboratory Evaluations in Molecular Medicine: Nutrients, Toxicants, and Cell Regulators, 2d edition* (Metametrix: Norcross, GA, 2007).

The authors would also like to pay special tribute to those incredible individuals who have pioneered this medicine: Archibald Garrod, MD, who first elucidated the concept of biochemical individuality in a 1902 article in the journal *Lancet*; Roger Williams, PhD, who popularized the term biochemical individuality in his 1956 book on the topic; Linus Pauling, PhD, a two-time Nobel Prize-winning scientist; Abram Hoffer, MD, who helped create the field of orthomolecular medicine with Dr. Pauling; Jeffrey Bland, PhD, who founded the Institute for Functional Medicine; Joseph Pizzorno, ND, founder of Bastyr University, avid proponent of science-based, natural medicine, and brilliant man who continually strives to understand the biochemical bases of health and disease; William Mitchell, ND, a co-founder of Bastyr University who inspired Dr. Neustadt to write this book; and many others. Their vision and desire for truly individualized medicine based on biochemical laws and uniqueness created a body of knowledge that has already begun to shift the medical paradigm in this country. We hope to move this revolution into mainstream medicine.

Introduction

The major purpose of this book is to declare a revolution in medical knowledge. We can no longer afford to deal with symptoms and medications that do not correspond to anything but arbitrary markers and theoretical suppositions about causations. The authors contend that all health, diseases, and cures are derived from three simple premises:

1: All health problems and diseases are biochemical.

2: If someone was healthy and he or she is not now, something has changed in his or her biochemistry.

3: If you treat the underlying biochemical dysfunction(s), you can prevent and cure disease.

Each of the premises, as simple as they may appear, combines centuries of clinical observation and deductions with contemporary biomedical research. The concept that health is a delicate balance between destructive and constructive forces, or as we call it in medicine, *catabolic* (destructive) and *anabolic* (constructive), has been around since at least the time of ancient Egypt and China. In Chinese medicine, this delicate balance is referred to as *yin* and *yang*.

The oldest medical systems in the world extensively used plants as medicine. In fact, the majority of the world's population to this day still turns to botanical medicines before they reach for pharmaceuticals. Throughout the ages, humans have relied on nature to supply the materials they need for their basic needs—for the production of foodstuffs, shelters, clothing, means of transportation, fertilizers, flavors, fragrances, and medicines. Plants have formed the basis of sophisticated traditional medical systems that have been in existence for thousands of years and continue to provide the world with new remedies. Botanical medicine is based on empirical findings over thousands of years, and although some of the therapeutic properties attributed to plants have been proven false, modern clinical research supports the use of plant medicines more often than not.

The first records of botanical medicines, written on clay tablets in cuneiform, are from Mesopotamia and date from about 2600 BC; among the substances that were used were oils of *Cedrus* species (cedar) and *Cupressus sempervirens* (cypress), *Glycyrrhiza glabra* (licorice), *Commiphora* species (myrrh), and *Papaver somniferum* (poppy juice), all of which are still used today for the treatment of ailments ranging from coughs and colds to parasitic infections and inflammation.[1]

The rise of the pharmaceutical industry in the United States did not begin until the twentieth century. The industry started during World War I and really took off after World War II. The premise of pharmaceutical companies' business model is that through the use of chemical processes, which in themselves are toxic, drugs can be created from natural products by isolating and concentrating specific elements of those natural substances. Using the isolated chemical or chemicals from plants and fungi, they can then cure diseases by literally providing a drug for the symptoms themselves. For example, antidepressant medications merely alleviate the symptoms of depression but do not cure depression.

The fundamental concept the reader can take away from this is that the pharmaceutical industry bases its actions on the goal of destroying cells or suppressing symptoms. The authors do not outright condemn this approach, but it is overused and has been implemented as the only legitimate approach taught in conventional medical schools. *Allopathic* medical systems, upon which conventional medicine is based, maintain that disease comes from outside the body. This is in contrast to the *nutritional biochemistry* approach whereby symptoms of disease are viewed as manifestations of biochemical dysfunctions that can largely be identified and corrected to support and promote health. This concept is taught in naturopathic medical schools, which may serve as the foundation for a truly integrative medical education system.

For example, antibiotics are overused to the extent that there is serious concern in the medical community that bacterial resistance to antibiotics is growing. This may cause an epidemic that no antibiotic can cure. This is true for *Streptococcus* (Strep throat), *Staphylococcus* and tuberculosis. However, not everyone who is exposed to these bacteria gets sick. Those who do not get sick have strong immune systems while those who do get sick have weaker immune systems. The nutrients and lifestyles required to produce a healthy immune system are well known, and providing the body what it needs to function better is the nutritional biochemistry approach. ·

Similarly, allopathic medicine prescribes antidepressants for many different conditions, even those that are not psychiatric in nature. These antidepressants include Prozac even though no one has a deficiency in Prozac. People may have deficiencies in essential amino acids, vitamins, minerals, and fatty acids.

Through biochemical testing, these can all be tested for and corrected with customized treatment plans aimed at improving biochemical function.

The emphasis of this book is to describe for the first time the legitimate use of biochemical testing in clinical practice for the consumer audience. Ironically, it is the reader, as a lay person, who will be more open to this information than physicians because many readers will have found that visiting an endless series of doctors, who have limited time and understanding of their symptoms and diseases, is extremely frustrating and detrimental to their health. It's not uncommon to hear complaints from people that they're frustrated that their doctors don't provide adequate service to them.

One specific case involved a twenty-five-year-old man who had complained for years to his physicians of abdominal pain, joint pain, swollen lymph nodes, and fatigue. All these symptoms were getting progressively worse. He had seen a family-practice doctor, allergy specialist, internist, and gastroenterologist. All of them were board certified in their respective specialties. The patient was rarely given time by his doctors to adequately explain his health history, and, when he did, the physicians were incapable of looking at it holistically or through any paradigm other than what they learned for their specialties. In other words, the patient was viewed through the biases and myopic vision of the medical specialists, which is prevalent throughout our entire medical system. All the physicians were incorrect in their diagnoses, and, when the patient did not improve under their care, each of them in turn simply suggested his problems stemmed from stress, anxiety, and depression, and that he should take antidepressant medications. The authors call this the "garbage can diagnosis," which is often given to patients when doctors don't understand the body's underlying biochemistry and fundamental medical issues.

When the authors of this book evaluated him, it was clear to them that he was suffering from multiple biochemical dysfunctions and malnutrition that were made worse by unnecessary medications and stomach surgery. Even after the authors successfully treated him with nutritional compounds based on his laboratory results and medical history, his primary physician refused to accept the notion that he was suffering from anything other than stress.

As this case clearly demonstrates, the science of using the body's own biochemistry to promote health is extremely powerful. It's important for the reader to understand that the authors are not simply practicing botanical or nutritional medicine, but they are integrating the best of conventional medicine with complementary biochemical medicine using the most advanced analytical tools.

This approach is so comprehensive that the testing requires seven vials of blood and one to two vials of urine. The testing of more than four hundred variables generates a report that is longer than forty pages. From this data, customized treatment plans are created to correct the underlying biochemical problems detected in the laboratory tests. Just as no two people are exactly alike, every treatment plan is unique. Patients are prescribed the highest-quality nutritional products formulated by the authors to target specific biochemical abnormalities detected in the laboratory tests. Their formulas are manufactured in an FDA-approved facility to the highest industry standards, and they pay extra to have all batches third-party tested for purity and potency.

Another crucial element of this revolution is the authors' focus on the particular compartment in cells called *mitochondria*. Mitochondria are the powerhouses of our cells. Among other functions, they are responsible for generating energy as adenosine triphosphate (ATP) and heat. Damage to mitochondria is implicated in every known disease, and it is discussed in greater detail in chapter five. The point here is that medicine has ignored the years of basic research showing that the biochemical pathways in cells can be evaluated and modulated using nutrients. Even supposed experts in mitochondrial disease, who use biopsies and electron scanning microscopy to evaluate mitochondria, are missing the point. These tests evaluate tissue that has been removed from the body, and, unfortunately, this is the standard in conventional medicine. When tissue is removed from the body and chemicals applied to it, the tissue is dead. The analysis is a structural one and not a functional one. Although the structure has been determined, it doesn't provide information about how the cells are functioning or how to treat them. A functional approach that analyzes the person's biochemistry can instead evaluate the biochemical pathways, which can then be improved with targeted nutritional therapies.

It is the authors' hope that people reading this book will understand that they or their loved ones do not need to continue suffering. Through an evaluation of the underlying biochemical pathways, this revolutionary approach in medicine offers hope and cures to millions. It is also their goal that the conventional medical system begins to teach and implement this approach so that the great health care burden, both physical and financial, can be reduced. The crisis in medicine is due largely to the ever-increasing number of people suffering from chronic, degenerative diseases for which allopathic medicine has very few effective treatments. The health care crisis stems directly from the fact that the philosophy underlying allopathic medicine is fundamentally incorrect. Nutritional biochemistry provides a realistic and proven solution to this crisis.

CHAPTER ONE

Why This Book Was Written

In 2006, a sixty-two-year-old man walked into Dr. Neustadt's clinic, Montana Integrative Medicine, (www.montanaim.com) in Bozeman, Montana. This gentleman, Steve Pieczenik, MD, PhD, (www.stevepieczenik.com) was complaining of shortness of breath, tightness in his chest, and an inability to exercise or walk long distances. Three months prior, Dr. Pieczenik was tested by a cardiologist and then a pulmonologist. The cardiologist found nothing wrong with his heart. The pulmonologist found a 22% deficit in oxygen intake and blood perfusion (decreased blood oxygen content). Neither of these physicians understood why this deficit was occurring, but both agreed that the bronchi in Dr. Pieczenik's lungs were constricting due to unspecified allergies. Dr. Pieczenik, however, had no history of any allergies. The solution offered, even though the doctors could not determine the underlying cause, was to prescribe steroids and an inhaler. This approach only treated his symptoms.

Since steroids and inhalers have been the most common therapy for these symptoms for many years, Dr. Pieczenik asked his doctors, "How come the treatment of exertion asthma has not changed in forty years?" Dr. Pieczenik, who is a medical doctor himself, was educated at Cornell University Medical School, Harvard Medical College, and MIT, and was a board examiner in psychiatry and neurology. Dr. Pieczenik did not accept the answers he was given because he felt that neither doctor understood the underlying causes of the problem. His diagnosis was relegated to the wastebasket of medicine—"the chronic, we-don't-really-understand-why catchall diagnosis." So, in turn, the catchall treatment was to prescribe steroids, which are handed out as though they are candy. Nevertheless, Dr. Pieczenik tried the steroids and inhaler and found them totally ineffectual, as he had expected. In fact, when he took the steroids, they kept him awake for more than seventy-two hours, a documented side effect of these drugs. Unfortunately, his physicians neglected to tell him of this side effect.

Dr. Pieczenik had no further medical solutions other than to search for a new paradigm in health, which he had done in other fields such as psychiatry (i.e., integrating political science and psychiatry). Dr. Pieczenik realized medicine had no solution to this particular problem and many other chronic diseases. He was fully aware that most diseases were merely treated with medications that decreased symptoms but did nothing to address the underlying causes. Also, as Dr. Pieczenik experienced with the steroids, many medications have dangerous side effects. He found that the practice of medicine had not really changed in over forty years, despite what was considered intensive research in genomics and molecular biology. By and large, from his point of view, medicine had reached a major impasse and had failed repeatedly.

By chance, Dr. Pieczenik met Dr. Neustadt, a naturopathic physician with a specialization in nutritional biochemistry, a couple of years earlier at Sweet Pea Festival, an annual summer arts and food festival in Bozeman. At that time, Dr. Pieczenik mentioned to Dr. Neustadt that he had a breathing difficulty that had not existed earlier in his life, and Dr. Neustadt casually said that Dr. Pieczenik probably had a decrease in epinephrine production. Epinephrine is a chemical in the body that, among other things, helps to dilate the lungs so people can breathe. Still skeptical of Dr. Neustadt's explanation, Dr. Pieczenik continued to endure his condition until one day he made an appointment with Dr. Neustadt and agreed to a comprehensive biochemical evaluation. His work-up included a standard medical evaluation with a physical examination, but Dr. Neustadt also ordered a series of blood and urine tests to analyze more than four hundred variables of biochemical function.

When the results came back, they showed that Dr. Pieczenik indeed had low epinephrine, and the specific reason was low copper amounts in his body. The simple explanation is that in order to produce epinephrine, we all need a combination of the raw materials required for it, which are amino acids, vitamins, and minerals. Specifically, the pathway for the production of epinephrine (see figure 1.1) requires the amino acid phenylalanine from diet, vitamin B3 (niacin), iron, biopterene, vitamin B6 (pyridoxine), vitamin C, copper, vitamin B12, and S-adenosyl methionine (SAMe). Additionally, since biochemistry is a web of interactions—and individual vitamins, minerals, and amino acids have multiple functions in the body—many other symptoms are associated with low levels of epinephrine and the other amino acids in this pathway (see table 1.1).

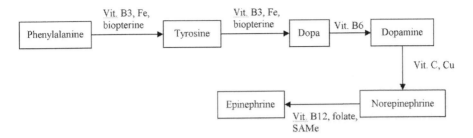

Figure 1.1. Pathway for the production of epinephrine, which is required for proper breathing. Abbreviations: Cu = copper, B3 = niacin, B6 = pyridoxine, Fe = iron, SAMe = S-adenosyl methionine, Vit. C = vitamin C.

In addition to the low copper, which directly explained his poor breathing, Dr. Pieczenik had low levels of some B-vitamins and had been getting too much zinc. What astonished Dr. Pieczenik was that he had been taking well-known brands of dietary supplements, including GNC, Nature's Way, Centrum, and Kirkland. The formulas he was taking, however, contained nutrient doses that were too low. They also contained nutrients in forms that were essentially not absorbable. For example, his dietary supplements contained magnesium as magnesium oxide. People can only absorb about 2% of this form of magnesium. It is so poorly absorbed that it is used clinically in higher dosages as a laxative for constipation. So if a dietary supplement contains one hundred milligrams of magnesium as magnesium oxide, people taking the dietary supplement are really only absorbing about two milligrams of magnesium. The same holds true for zinc and copper in their oxide forms, which he was taking.

Table 1.1. Low amino acids and their symptoms[2-6]

Low	Symptoms
Tyrosine	Brain fog Fatigue Feeling frequently cold Increased cholesterol Weight gain
Dopamine	Depression Seizures

Epinephrine	Allergies
	Anorexia
	Apathy
	Asthma and exertion-onset breathing difficulties
	Chronic pain
	Fatigue/malaise
	Inability to cope
	Myocardial infarction (heart attack)
	Reduced libido
	Restless sleep
	Risk of autoimmune disease
	Risk of inflammatory conditions
	Unable to perform routine tasks
	Weakness

Moreover, the tests also identified that he had a major fungal infection in the bowels in the same location that his mother had cancer, from which she died. Similarly, he also had elevated insulin, a hormone required for proper utilization of blood sugar, which indicated a risk of developing diabetes. This was a complete surprise again to Dr. Pieczenik since his fasting blood sugar level, which is the standard medical test for diabetes screening, had always been normal. Additionally, it turned out that several members of his family had developed mature-onset diabetes, which meant Dr. Pieczenik was at a higher risk of developing it simply due to his family history.

In other words, here was a well-known, board-certified physician who had received the most sophisticated conventional medical evaluations in the country and was still unable to discover the underlying problems putting him at risk for diabetes, heart attack, cancer, and premature death. As a typical board examiner, he asked himself, "What was wrong with the patient? What conditions could result in his shortness of breath other than a heart condition and mature-onset asthma secondary to an allergen?" After mulling over the problem, he felt that he was lacking the correct paradigm to sufficiently diagnose his own problem and answer his own questions.

For Dr. Neustadt, this was a simple textbook case because of his extensive experience in biochemical medicine. Dr. Neustadt understood that all symptoms are manifestations of biochemical dysfunction. That is, if a person was not sick last year, or yesterday, and today he or she is sick, then something has changed in his or her biochemistry. By testing a person's biochemistry, the problematic pathways may be identified and corrected using nutritional medicine. When the pathways are corrected, health is promoted and a cure is possible.

Dr. Neustadt prescribed diet and nutrients to correct Dr. Pieczenik's biochemical abnormalities. Dr. Pieczenik's copper level was corrected, and all of his breathing difficulties resolved within two weeks. He was prescribed a proper nutritional and exercise program to help him lose weight and decrease his high insulin and risk of diabetes, while the fungal infection in his bowels was treated to decrease his colorectal cancer risk. Upon follow-up testing, all of his parameters were normal. But even more immediately important to him than his laboratory values was the fact that he could breath again. In fact, Dr. Pieczenik was able to live through Montana's raging fires and the poor air quality during the summer of 2006 without any breathing difficulties. Normally, he would have evacuated to the East Coast.

Dr. Pieczenik realized through his own experience that this new concept in medicine must reach a larger audience. This compelled him to create another company, on top of the thirty other successful companies that he had already founded, to unify his expertise with Dr. Neustadt's unique approach to diagnosing and treating diseases. In the summer of 2006, Drs. Pieczenik and Neustadt founded Nutritional Biochemistry, Inc., (NBI) and NBI Testing and Consulting Corporation. These companies focus on the testing and analysis of clinically relevant biochemical pathways and the treatment of abnormal pathways using medical nutrition. Through a combination of blood and urine samples, more than four hundred biochemical parameters can be evaluated and corrected so as to promote a person's health instead of simply treating symptoms.

The authors wrote this book in response to the extensive requests by people who had been helped by Montana Integrative Medicine, NBI, and NBI Testing and Consulting Corporation. They asked Drs. Neustadt and Pieczenik to write a book so that they could share this information with their friends, families, and colleagues. Doctors (medical, naturopathic, chiropractic, osteopathic) all over the world have contacted Drs. Pieczenik and Neustadt asking how they can implement this powerful approach in their practices. In the winter of 2007, Drs. Pieczenik and Neustadt began writing this book, and they decided to self-publish it so it could be in readers' hands in the shortest amount of time. Without trying to be overly dramatic, they felt that every moment that passed without publishing this knowledge, another person was misdiagnosed and mistreated, with sometimes fatal consequences.

It is their sincere hope that this book begins a medical revolution in which diseases are evaluated properly, with causes identified and treated, and stops the tendency to throw more and more drugs at ever-worsening symptoms, a corrupt healthcare model that the pharmaceutical companies have a vested interest in creating and maintaining.

Drs. Neustadt and Pieczenik wish readers an enjoyable introduction to this new way of looking at their own bodies. Please do not worry if some of the concepts initially seem complicated. The basic premise, as stated above, is that all disease is biochemical, and correcting the underlying biochemistry promotes health. If people only understand this one concept, then they have grasped the entire essence of this book.

Both doctors hope that this information helps you or someone you love to improve their health.

CHAPTER TWO

Are Dietary Supplements Dangerous?

In 2004, a study was published in the journal *Annals of Internal Medicine*. The authors concluded that taking vitamin E supplements can increase one's risk of dying.[7] More recently, the *Journal of the American Medical Association (JAMA)* published an article that concluded taking antioxidant vitamins can also increase the risk of death.[8] These two studies are called *meta-analyses*, which means they combined data from many different studies and analyzed the pooled data. The premise behind a meta-analysis is that if you can increase the number of study participants by combining different studies, you can draw a more accurate conclusion. Two major criteria, however, must be met for the results of a meta-analysis to be valid. First, the participants in the different clinical trials must be similar with respect to age and medical conditions. Second, the study medications, dosages, and protocols must be similar. Neither of these studies complied with even these basic criteria.

A meta-analysis is only as strong as the data combined for analysis. Randomized, controlled trials are done on different populations and subgroups representing various patient characteristics. Since diverse subgroups may respond to the same therapy differently, combining very heterogeneous studies can make the analysis unreliable.[9] A meta-analysis should analyze data from homogenous populations using similar study protocols. Not only did these meta-analyses not meet these criteria for a high-quality study, their conclusions conflict with prior meta-analyses on the health benefits of these nutrients.

The short answer to the question as to whether dietary supplements are safe is an overwhelming yes. One major reason why the dietary supplement industry is not regulated more strictly is because the safety profile of dietary supplements is excellent. The pharmaceutical model of health care creates drugs that take over the body's biochemical function instead of working with the body's biochemistry to promote health. The number of dangerous side effects mentioned during medication commercials frequently strikes people as alarming. Many times these side effects are quite dangerous and can be lethal.

In contrast, a review of the clinical trials into the use of nutrients reveals that the vast majority of adverse effects are minor and temporary. Whereas medications more often than not carry the risk of dangerous side effects, dietary supplements usually carry the risk of *side benefits*, which is a term the authors created to describe the potential indirect benefits to using nutrients in addition the direct benefits that are being targeted clinically.

A striking illustration of side benefits involved a sixty-year-old Vietnam veteran who was suffering from extreme fatigue and photophobia (sensitivity to light). When he awoke in the morning, his energy would be good, but he had to nap every three hours during the day because his energy would diminish to nothing. While in the clinic, he requested the window shades be drawn because of his extreme sensitivity to light. Biochemical testing revealed several abnormalities in his energy-producing pathways, amino-acid deficiencies, free-radical damage to his DNA (a risk factor for cancer), problems with his liver-detoxification pathways, and an intestinal bacterial infection. His major complaint was extreme fatigue, and the treatment plan was tailored to correct his biochemical abnormalities to provide more energy. One month later, he returned and only had to nap once a day. To his surprise, his light sensitivity had also greatly improved. The window blinds did not have to be drawn, and his wife reported that he had enough energy to start riding his motorcycle again.

The problem is that many people who object to using nutrients clinically are simply unfamiliar with the basic research and clinical trials supporting its use. The National Institute of Health (NIH) manages the nation's largest database of peer-reviewed scholarly journals, which can be accessed at www.pubmed.com. There are more than six million entries in its database, which is a phenomenal amount of research. A search for all studies on the amino acid carnitine yields more than nine thousand entries and a search for vitamin C returns over twelve thousand entries. It is the authors' assertion that those who state that research does not support the use of nutrients in clinical practice have simply not done their homework.

CHAPTER THREE

Your Body,
Your Biochemistry

Biochemistry is the process by which your body uses nutrients to function. These nutrients are amino acids, vitamins, and minerals. This process entails a web of interactions among biochemical pathways and body systems. Since biochemistry is a web of interactions, the most effective approach is a holistic medical intake combined with comprehensive biochemical testing that allows skilled clinicians to connect the dots between seemingly disparate symptoms. This chapter introduces basic concepts in biochemistry and nutrition that are used throughout the rest of the book when discussing diseases, biochemical tests, and treatment options.

Amino Acids

Amino acids are composed simply of carbon, oxygen, hydrogen, nitrogen, and sometimes sulfur. They are the building blocks of proteins. Proteins contain multiple amino acids strung together like letters of an alphabet. These letters (amino acids) can be combined in almost an infinite number of ways to produce the diversity of proteins seen in humans.

People produce about five hundred thousand different proteins, which act as hormones to control mood, energy, and appetite; connective tissue such as skin, hair, and nails; and muscles.[10] For example, phenylalanine is an amino acid. Phenylalanine, as shown in figure 1.1, travels down its pathway to produce tyrosine, dopamine, and epinephrine. It also produces niacin (vitamin B3), thyroid hormones, and melanin, a skin pigment.[11]

You may see phenylalanine sometimes on a food or dietary supplement label with the warning, "Phenylketonurics—contains phenylalanine." Phenylketonuria (PKU) is disorder is screened for at birth and has an incidence of 1 in 10,000. People with this condition have difficulty transforming phenylalanine to tyrosine. Phenylalanine therefore accumulates in the blood and causes mental and physical retardation.

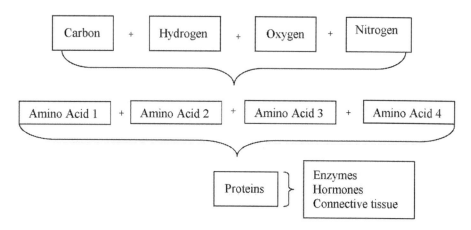

Figure 2.1. Raw materials such as carbon, hydrogen, oxygen, and nitrogen are combined to create amino acids, which join together to create proteins. Proteins function in our bodies as hormones, enzymes, and connective tissue.

Phenylalanine is found in all protein foods, and neonates diagnosed with this condition are placed on a phenylalanine-restricted diet and supplemented with tyrosine, vitamins, minerals, and other amino acids. While effective, maintaining this severely limited diet is quite difficult in school-age children, it leads to socially awkward situations for adults, and it is complicated in pregnant women. Fortunately, as you will discover reading this book, the problem in people with phenylketonuria is simply a problem with inefficient transformation of phenylalanine to tyrosine. The enzyme (protein that facilitates a biochemical reaction) that converts phenylalanine to tyrosine in many people with PKU still functions, although inefficiently.

Since 1999, several clinical trials have reported positive results in decreasing serum phenylalanine in people with this condition by administering pharmacological doses of tetrahydrobiopterin (BH_4), a nutrient required for this enzyme to function. In one small study involving five children, serum phenylalanine concentrations declined in four of five of them with a loading dose of ten milligrams of BH_4 per kilogram body weight.[12] A larger study conducted in 2002 showed that BH_4 significantly lowered phenylalanine in 87% of the children by as much as 92%.[13] Infants and children with this disorder should now also be tested for their responsiveness to BH_4 therapy, as it may allow many of them to consume a less restrictive diet and some to even cease the therapeutic diet altogether.

What this study showed is that even in seemingly severe genetic conditions, there may be some enzyme activity that can be stimulated with pharmaco-logic dosages of nutrients, and diseases once viewed as incurable may in fact be ameliorated with nutrients. This study also reminds the authors of an observation by Roger Williams, PhD, in 1956, when he wrote, "Whenever an extreme genetic character appears in an individual organism, it should be taken as an indication (unless there is proof to the contrary) that less extreme and gradu-ated genetic characters of the same sort exist in other individual organisms."[14]

Vitamins

Vitamins are nutrients required for essential metabolic reactions in the body. Vitamins are divided into two general categories—fat-soluble and water-solu-ble. The fat-soluble group includes vitamin A, D, K, and E.[15] Fat-soluble vita-mins are better absorbed when ingested with some fat and can be stored in fat within the body. The reason why fat-soluble vitamins are absorbed more effec-tively when you consume them with additional fat, as with a meal, is because fat causes the excretion of bile into the small intestines from the gallbladder. The bile surrounds the fat and makes it more absorbable by the small intes-tines. Fat-soluble vitamins can be stored in tissues, meaning that there is a risk for toxicity. For example, high dosages of vitamin A can cause liver damage in children and adults, and in pregnant women it can cause damage to fetuses.[16]

Water-soluble vitamins include the B-complex vitamins—B1 (thiamin), B2 (riboflavin), B3 (niacin), B5 (pantothenic acid), B6 (pyridoxine), B12 (cobala-min) folic acid, and biotin—as well as vitamin C (ascorbic acid).[15] Water-sol-uble vitamins do not need fat for absorption, and they also carry a much lower risk for toxicity. Water-soluble vitamins are not stored in fat and are excreted in the urine. The only water-soluble vitamins that carry any appreciable risk for toxicity are vitamins B3 and B6. If you get too much of the other water-soluble vitamins, you simply urinate them out. Vitamin B2 may cause a harm-less yellowish-green discoloration to the urine.

Patients frequently ask whether or not they are absorbing the vitamins since they see their urine change color. They believe, and have heard, that people shouldn't take high doses of the water-soluble vitamins because they don't absorb them. The simple answer is yes; they are absorbing them. In order for vitamins to appear in urine, people must absorb them through the intestines, where they enter the blood stream, circulate through the body, and bathe cells with their nutrients prior to appearing in the urine. The cells will extract from the blood the amounts they need, and the excess appears in the urine.

The amount of these vitamins the body needs depends on many factors, including diet, stress, and ongoing infections. For example, one of the places in the body where vitamin C is most concentrated is in white blood cells.[17] These cells comprise our immune system that protects us from bacteria and viruses. When people get a cold or flu, their bodies' ability to absorb vitamin C from the bowels increases. That is, they find that when they're sick they absorb up to tens times more vitamin C than when they're healthy.[18] This reflects the body's ability to adapt to different situations that require different amounts of nutrients. To test this, people can do what's called the Bowel Tolerance Test.[18-20] "To bowel tolerance" means that they take ever-increasing amounts of vitamin C, such as one thousand milligrams every hour for one day, then two thousand milligrams every hour for the next day, and so on, until their intestines cannot absorb anymore. When this happens, they may experience some burning, loose stools, or watery diarrhea when they have a bowel movement. This signals that they've reached bowel tolerance and need to decrease the amount taken to the dose at which these discomforts did not appear. Bowel tolerance can vary from person to person, and can be as low as one thousand milligrams per day when healthy and greater than ten thousand milligrams per day when sick.

Minerals

Examples of minerals include calcium, magnesium, manganese, copper, zinc, selenium, iron, and vanadium. Except for calcium, which concentrates outside of cells, all other minerals are pumped into cells where they concentrate and do their work. For example, magnesium, which is required for more than three hundred biochemical reactions in the body, concentrates in cells where it is required for the generation of cellular energy, called adenosine triphosphate (ATP).[21] Muscles also use magnesium to allow them to relax after a contraction, thereby explaining why a low magnesium level sometimes manifests itself as muscle cramps. Unfortunately, conventional medical labs only measure magnesium in the serum (the liquid portion of blood) and not intracellular magnesium, which gives a false impression that someone has normal magnesium when, in fact, their intracellular magnesium may be low. Many people have a deficiency in intracellular magnesium, since it's been estimated that 56% of people do not eat the recommended daily value of magnesium.[22] Additionally, magnesium deficiency can cause DNA damage and may contribute to the development of cancer.[22]

Selenium is used in the body for many different functions. One of its functions is to produce active thyroid hormone, T3, from the conversion of the inactive thyroid hormone, T4, in different tissues in the body.[23, 24] This conversion also requires zinc.[25] This is important because symptoms of low thyroid function include fatigue, depression, weight gain, and low body temperature. Low thyroid function can also cause increased cholesterol, a risk factor for heart disease and stroke.[26] However, conventional screening tests for thyroid function do not test for the actual thyroid hormones themselves or for selenium and zinc. Instead, the standard screening test for low thyroid function, called hypothyroidism, is a measurement of thyroid-stimulating hormone (TSH). TSH is actually produced in a region of the brain called the anterior pituitary gland, and its role is to stimulate the production T4 and T3 by the thyroid gland, which is located in the lower end of a person's neck. Doctors find that people can have "functional hypothyroidism," which means that their TSH and T4 levels are normal, but their T3 is low. People who only receive the conventional medical workup can experience depression, fatigue, difficulty losing weight, and frequent coldness when the underlying cause may be low thyroid function because of low selenium or zinc.

Non-Vitamin Nutrients

In addition to the vitamins listed above, there are nutrients derived from plants, called *phytonutrients* (*phyto* means plant in Greek), which have specific beneficial properties. One class of these compounds, called *flavonoids*, are powerful antioxidants.[27] An antioxidant "quenches" free radicals, which are unstable molecules that damage proteins, DNA, and cell membranes. A urine test measures free-radical damage to DNA, which is a risk factor for cancer.[22] Free-radical damage to lipids (fats)is a risk factor for heart disease, and a blood test measures this condition.[28-32] Free radicals are produced naturally as the byproducts of cellular processes, such as the production of cellular energy.[33] Additionally, free radicals make up a vital component of the immune system since they are produced by white blood cells to kill viruses and bacteria.[34]

Like everything in life, balance is the key. The body needs a certain amount of free radicals to function properly, but excessive free radicals cause diseases. Antioxidants keep free radicals in balance. These antioxidant molecules include flavonoids, vitamins A, C, and E, glutathione, alpha lipoic acid, and many others. They can donate an electron that neutralizes the free radical. By quenching free radicals, antioxidants stop them from doing additional damage to other molecules.

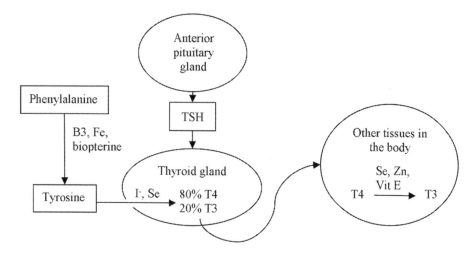

Figure 2.2 Pathway and nutrients necessary for proper thyroid hormone production.

Flavonoids are found in high amounts in darkly pigmented fruits such as blueberries, blackberries, plums, and cherries; and also in vegetables. Flavonoids are more powerful antioxidants than vitamin C, and they can help increase the strength of blood vessels, decrease inflammation, and lower the risks for cancer and cardiovascular diseases.[35-42] Table 2.2 lists some flavonoids and the plants in which they're found. Frequently, the advice given to patients is to "eat a rainbow a day" of fruits and vegetables, meaning that people should eat a variety of differently colored, fresh whole fruits and vegetables each day to ensure an ample supply of phytonutrients. Additionally, when fresh fruit is not available, it can be helpful to purchase frozen fruits, such as cherries or blueberries, and eat a cup a day of frozen fruit.

Table 2.2. Plant-derived antioxidants, their roles in the body, and sources[43]

Antioxidant	Description	Good Sources
Beta-carotene	Precursor to vitamin A	Yellow, orange, and green leafy fruits and vegetables (e.g., carrots, spinach, lettuce, tomatoes, sweet potatoes, broccoli, cantaloupe, winter squash).

Caffeic acid	A carboxylic acid found in many fruits, vegetables, seasonings, and beverages	Dandelion (*Taraxacum officinale*), Yarrow (*Achillea millefolium*), Horsetail (*Equisetum arvense*, among others)
Curcumin	A polyphenol that is the active ingredient of the spice turmeric and is yellow when isolated; a powerful anti-inflammatory compound	Turmeric (*Curcuma longa*) root
Epigallocatechin gallate (EGCG)	A catechin (class of tannins) with antioxidant activity about 25-100 times that of vitamins C and E	Green tea
Genistein	An isoflavone (class of flavonoids) with phytoestrogenic activities	Soybeans and soy foods
Kaempferol	A flavonoid that is yellow when isolated	Apples, onions, leeks, citrus fruits, grapes, red wine, *Gingko biloba*, St. John's wort (*Hypericum perforatum*)
Quercetin	A flavonoid	Apples, black tea, green tea, onions, raspberries, red wine, red grapes, citrus fruits, broccoli, leafy green vegetables, cherries
Resveratrol	A polyphenolic phytoalexin produced by plants as an antinfungal agent.	Skin of red grapes
Silymarin	A mixture of flavolignans (silybinin, silidianin, silicristin) that increases endogenous glutathione	Milk thistle (*Silybum marianum*)

Fats

While many people believe low-fat diets are healthy, the fact is that our bodies require fats for proper function. Fats make up 60% of the brain and central nervous system. The membranes that surround every cell are comprised of two layers of fats, called the *lipid bilayer*. These fats are involved in communication between cells and the production of hormones and other vital chemicals.

There are different classes of fats, including saturated and unsaturated fatty acids. The unsaturated fatty acids are further defined as omega-6 and omega-3 fatty acids. Modern diets that are high in animal meats are high in omega-6 fats and low in omega-3 fats. Omega-6 fatty acids can contribute to chronic degenerative diseases and promote inflammation. High amounts of omega-3 fatty acids are found in fish and plants, and they are considered anti-inflammatory and protective against some chronic, degenerative diseases such as cardiovascular disease. Saturated fats, another class of fatty acids, are found in beef and other land animals and can contribute to heart disease. Unsaturated fatty acids are liquid at room temperature while saturated fatty acids are solid at room temperature.

Diet and Nutrients

A discussion of nutrients would be incomplete without mentioning the role proper nutrition plays in our health. Food contains the vital nutrients required for our bodies to function, but there are several reasons why most people become deficient in nutrients as they age. One simple reason is that people do not eat an optimal diet. The Mediterranean Dietary Pattern has been studied for more than thirty years and has been shown repeatedly to reduce the risk of cancer, diabetes, cardiovascular disease, obesity, and premature death.[44, 45] This diet is essentially the opposite of the Standard American Diet (SAD) that promotes cancer, diabetes, cardiovascular disease, obesity, and premature death.[46-49] The SAD diet is propagated by multi-million dollar advertising campaigns that convince people that eating processed foods and high amounts of beef is necessary and beneficial. This in fact is completely false. The Mediterranean Diet is a whole-foods, plant-based diet that stresses consuming whole grains, whole fruits and vegetables, and fish. It is low in saturated fat and high in fiber from complex carbohydrates.

Meat consumption in the Mediterranean Diet is monthly, while people following a SAD pattern of eating consume red meat multiple times each week. In most parts of the United States, this means eating farm-raised beef that was finished on corn and treated throughout its life with hormones and antibiotics. In contrast, wild game and meat that is hormone free, antibiotic free, and grass fed and grass finished contains a healthier profile of fatty acids than conventional meats.

Fatty acids surround every cell in our bodies and are crucial for proper cell functions. There are two major classes of fatty acids—omega-3 fatty acids and omega-6 fatty acids. Omega-3 fatty acids are anti-inflammatory, while omega-6 fatty acids promote inflammation and heart disease. Omega-3 fatty acids are found in high amounts in plant oils and cold-water fish, while meats (e.g., beef) contain higher amounts of omega-6 fatty acids.[54-56]

Different concentrations of fatty acids exist in foods, and both omega-3 and omega-6 fatty acids are required for proper health. However, the SAD contains too much

A word about eggs

Eggs are excellent sources of protein and biotin, a water-soluble vitamin, and lutein and zeaxanthin, two fat-soluble vitamins that can help preserve eyesight. One egg contains approximately five grams of protein.

There is a misconception that eggs increase cholesterol. The fact is that ingestion of moderate amounts of eggs does not adversely affect lipid levels in the majority of patients. Instead, it is when eggshells are cracked and the yolk is scrambled that free radicals create problems. When egg whites and yolks are exposed to air and heat, such as when you make an omelet, the fats in the egg become rancid, and it's just like eating a wonderfully delicious meal of free radicals that enter your body and cause damage to your blood vessels and other cells. On the other hand, hard-boiled eggs are good for you and do not contain the free radicals found in scrambled or fried eggs because the shell in hard-boiled eggs is left intact; therefore the egg yolk and egg white are not exposed to oxygen.[50-53]

omega-6 fatty acid and too little omega-3 fatty acid.[47] This unfavorable ratio promotes inflammation and plays an important role in many diseases such as heart disease and dementia. In short, the SAD is comprised mostly of processed foods and red meat and is high in saturated fat, simple sugars, and trans fats, and it is low in fiber. For an excellent discussion of the science behind a whole-foods, plant based diet, we recommend readers pick up a copy of the book *The China Study*, by T. Colin Campbell, PhD, who has been researching the links between diet and cancer for more than forty years and is a Professor Emeritus of Nutritional Biochemistry at Cornell University.[57]

Many food products in the American diet are inherently low in vitamins and minerals. For example, the conventional agricultural system in the United States has depleted the soils of vitamins and minerals, which are then not available for the plants to take up from the soils. The result, which has been confirmed in multiple studies, is that conventionally grown foods are lower in vitamins and minerals compared to organically grown foods.[58]

Processed foods such as white rice, pasta, potato chips, and baked goods that use white flour are nearly devoid of vitamins and minerals (see table 2.3).[59, 60] These foods are consumed in large quantities in the United States and are a cause of nutritional deficiencies. For example, about 85% of magnesium and 60% of calcium are lost during the process of refining wheat to make white flour for breads, muffins, cookies, and pizza dough.[61, 62] The naturally occurring nutrients are stripped out during the processing of these foods by removing the most nutrient-dense portion of the grain and applying heat during the manufacturing process that destroys vitamins.

> ## A word about frozen versus fresh foods
>
> In some instances, frozen foods may actually be healthier than "fresh" fruits and vegetables. This has to do with one simple rule: the farther fruits and vegetables have to travel from the farm to your table, the longer they have to degrade and spoil. The moment a fruit or plant is detached from the soil, it stops taking up nutrients and begins the sometimes slow, sometimes rapid, process of decaying and dying. During this process, nutrients are depleted. Therefore, in instances where fresh fruits and vegetables from a nearby farm are not available, frozen fruits and vegetables may be more nutritious because the process of freezing locks in nutrients, as long as the food is not processed first (that is, heat is not applied).

These deficiencies set in motion dysfunctions in biochemical pathways that cause chronic, degenerative conditions such as cardiovascular disease, and they parallel the extremely common deficiencies detected by laboratory panels that test for vitamin and mineral deficiencies.[63]

Table 2.3. Percent of vitamin and mineral losses during the refining of flour

Vitamins	Lost (percent)
Vitamin B1 (thiamine)	77

Vitamin B2 (riboflavin)	80
Vitamin B3 (niacin)	81
Vitamin B5 (pantothine)	50
Vitamin B6 (pyridoxine)	72
Folic acid	67
Vitamin E	86
Betaine	23
Choline	30
Minerals	**Lost (percent)**
Calcium	60
Chromium	40
Copper	68
Iron	76
Magnesium	85
Manganese	86
Potassium	77
Selenium	16
Zinc	78

Digestion and Assimilation of Nutrients

Even when someone is eating an optimal diet, they may not be digesting and assimilating the nutrients properly. There are three major reasons for this. Someone's digestion may not be functioning properly; they may have food intolerances that cause chronic immune activation in the gut;[64-66] or they may have bacterial or fungal infections in the gut, called *intestinal dysbiosis*.[64, 67] Each of these situations can occur individually or together, and all result in putting one at risk for decreased ability to absorb nutrients.

Digestion involves the breakdown of large molecules into smaller, readily absorbed molecules. While some digestion begins with the production of enzymes in the mouth, the stomach is where the process of digestion really gets underway. Cells in the stomach excrete specific enzymes to break apart fats, starches, and proteins. The enzymes, however, are inactive and must be activated by stomach acid. When someone produces enough stomach acid, proper digestion in the stomach occurs. But many people don't produce enough stomach acid. Low stomach acid production is called *hypochlorhydria,* and when no stomach acid is produced it's called *achlorhydria.* Decreased stomach acid production occurs from aging, caffeine, overeating, stress, medications (especially those that block the production or excretion of stomach acid such as Protonix, Tagamet, Pepcid, Axid, Zantac, Prevacid, Prilosec, Aciphex, Nexium), alcohol, and stomach surgeries that destroy the acid-producing cells.

Many people produce less stomach acid as they age, and it's been estimated that 10–21% of people sixty to sixty-nine years old, 31% of those seventy to seventy-nine years old, and 37% of those above the age of eighty have hypochlorhydria or achlorhydria, and this rate may be higher in people with autoimmune conditions.[68, 69] One question posed to patients to screen for their risk of low stomach acid is, "Do you feel fuller sooner than you used to and stay full longer than you used to when you eat?" If the answer is yes, it may be that they have low stomach acid since decreased stomach acid increases the amount of time food sits in the stomach before passing into the small intestines. When stomach acid is low, vitamins and minerals may not be efficiently released from the food that contains them. This may result in decreased availability of nutrients for absorption and nutritional deficiencies. People with low stomach acid have been shown to be at increased risk for vitamin and mineral deficiencies.[70-74] Symptoms of low stomach acid production include bloating or distension after eating, diarrhea or constipation, flatulence after a meal, hair loss in women, heartburn, indigestion, malaise, and prolonged sense of fullness after eating.[74, 75] Additionally, the risk of hip fracture increases by 22% after one year and nearly 60% after four years in people taking acid-blocking medications as compared to people not taking them.[76]

Stomach acid plays two other important roles. It acts to sterilize food and signals the lower esophageal sphincter (the muscle separating the esophagus from the stomach) to close.[77-79] The gut normally contains about four hundred different species of bacteria, which are required for normal digestion and absorption of nutrients.[80, 81] It has been estimated that there are more bacterial cells in the gut than all the cells in the body combined.[82] These beneficial bacteria are required for normal digestion and absorption of nutrients. When inadequate sterilization of food occurs, however, pathogenic (bad) bacteria, viruses, and fungi can pass into the small intestines. This disrupts the healthy ecology in the gut and alters the delicate balance between healthy and unhealthy microbes. This imbalance in intestinal flora is called *dysbiosis,* and it can occur with the overgrowth of pathogenic bacteria and/or fungus. Symptoms of intestinal dysbiosis include abdominal gas and bloating, post-nasal drip, "brain fog" (feeling like you're just not mentally sharp), and sugar cravings.[63] Abdominal gas and bloating are caused by fermentation of food by the bacteria and fungus, which causes the production of gas, such as methane. Post-nasal drip is caused by immune system activation by bacteria and fungi. Sugar is the preferred energy source for the fungi, which can lead to sugar cravings. Bacteria and fungi secrete their own waste products, such as ammonia, that can enter the blood stream, cross into the brain, and cause brain fog. Additionally, intestinal bacterial overgrowth is now understood to be a risk factor for developing gastroesophageal reflux disorder (GERD).[83]

A simple urine test can detect acids secreted by pathogenic intestinal bacteria and fungi. These acids enter the blood stream, are filtered by the kidneys, and excreted in the urine. They include d-arabinitol, p-hydroxybenzoate, indican, tricarballylate and dihydroxyphenylpropionate.[63]

When low stomach acid production decreases the ability of the lower esophageal sphincter to close, the result is that the acid produced in the stomach can reflux up into the esophagus and cause symptoms of GERD.[84] The typical medical response to gastric reflux, which can cause burning, coughing, and asthma-like symptoms, is to prescribe acid-blocking medications. However, the actual cause in many people is too little acid and not too much acid.[84] Decreased acid production can occur as a result of decreased histidine, an amino acid that is required for acid secretion.[11] This amino acid is tested as part of an amino acid blood panel, which may diagnose the underlying cause in some patients. Stomach acid production can also be tested by using a meter, called a Heidelburg pH capsule test. Providing histidine to people with low stomach acid can improve their stomach acid production. Low stomach acid can also occur in from infections, such as *Helicobacter pylori* (*H. pylori*) in the stomach.[84] Additionally, when people have low stomach acid production, some doctors provide hydrochloric acid capsules for people to take with meals that help improve their digestion and eliminate GERD. There are some instances when people should not supplement with acid pills, and the authors of this book strongly advise people against supplementing with hydrochloric acid unless under the care of a doctor.

Food intolerances can also cause decreased absorption of nutrients by creating chronic inflammation in the intestines. Eighty percent of the immune system is clustered around the intestines.[85] When people repeatedly consume food that causes an immune activation in the gut, it creates intestinal irritation.[86] Over time, the cells lining the intestines become damaged. This can create malabsorption with decreased ability to assimilate nutrients from food. An extreme example of this is Celiac disease. Intolerance to wheat, rye, barley, and oats characterizes this disease. The immune system actually reacts to gluten contained in these foods. This causes intestinal inflammation and destruction of the cells lining the intestines. Celiac disease has wide-ranging symptoms, including fatigue, anemia, joint pains, depression, loss of balance, and malnutrition.[87, 88]

More frequently, people will react to foods that they crave, such as milk and eggs, which can be detected through a special blood test. This blood test is called an IgG food intolerance test, and people with rheumatoid arthritis, eczema, and other conditions have been shown to have elevated IgG antibodies to foods.[89, 90] IgG is a protein produced by the immune system. Most doctors only test for IgE-mediated allergies, which are also called "immediate hyper-sensitivity reactions." An IgE-mediated-immune response is responsible for the life-threatening reaction in some people to bee stings or peanuts. IgG, on the other hand, is a delayed-type-hypersensitivity reaction that, as the name implies, is not immediately apparent.[91] People who test negative on an IgE test can be positive on an IgG test.[92]

IgG reactions may take hours or days to appear, and symptoms can include post-nasal drip, gas and bloating, difficulty losing weight, joint aches, eczema, fatigue, and others. Food intolerances can cause these diverse symptoms for various reasons. Similar to bacterial and fungal dysbiosis, the immune-system activation caused by food intolerances can cause post-nasal drip. Gas and bloating is a result of incomplete digestion of food and the resultant fermentation of these food particles by bacteria in the intestines. Difficulty losing weight may result from an increased cortisol response by the body due to the continual stress placed on the immune system. When cortisol is chronically elevated, it causes an accumulation of abdominal fat.

The explanation for eczema and joint pains is a little more complicated. When the immune system in the intestines is activated, the antibody-antigen complexes enter the blood stream. An antibody is the protein produced by the immune system such as IgG, and an antigen is the molecule against which the immune system is reacting, such as a protein in milk. These antibody-antigen complexes travel from the intestines to the liver where they are broken down for elimination by the body. This process is like a conveyor belt where the antibody-antigen complexes are delivered to the liver for processing, but the amount of complexes delivered to the liver over time can overwhelm the liver's ability to detoxify them. When this occurs, the complexes pass through the liver and enter the systemic circulation. Like bits of sand in a river, these complexes can settle out of the blood stream where the flow of blood slows down. This occurs in the skin and joints. When these complexes are deposited in skin and joints, they act as irritants that can create local immune-system activation and produce such symptoms as joint pains and eczema. Frequently, the joint pains will be migratory, meaning different joints will be affected at different times.

Chronic stress predisposes people to low stomach acid production and food intolerances. This is because stress stimulates the release of cortisol, norepinephrine, and epinephrine. These are part of the *flight or flight* response to stress. The analogy that's often used to teach this concept to medical student is, "Imagine that you're being chased by a tiger." The body has two responses. It either flees or battles it out. In either case, cortisol and epinephrine are secreted to prepare people for action. They increase blood flow to skeletal muscles and decrease it to the intestines. These hormones also increase heart rate and alter blood flow in the brain. By shifting blood flow away from the intestines and to the muscles, digestion decreases. This can also cause damage to the cells lining the intestines and create a "hyperpermeable gut." When digestion decreases, it allows larger food particles to enter the small intestines where food is absorbed through the lining of the gut and into the body. The larger food particles, combined with the damaged lining of the gut, can activate the immune system and create food intolerances.

The fight or flight response is part of the sympathetic nervous system. Balancing the sympathetic arm of the nervous system is the parasympathetic nervous system. In contrast to the fight or flight response, the parasympathetic nervous system is referred to as the *rest and digest* response. If people slow down when they eat, and eat in a relaxed fashion, the sympathetic nervous system decreases activity and the parasympathetic nervous system increases activity. When this occurs, blood flows to the intestines for improved digestion and assimilation of nutrients. Taking time for relaxation is imperative for proper body function. Relaxation is vital for promoting health, and many people do not take any time out for this during their busy weeks.

Chapter Four

Kinetics

Kinetics in biochemistry is the study of how one molecule gets transformed into another molecule. For example, vitamin B6 is required for the production of dopamine from the enzyme DOPA decarboxylase.[93] Low dopamine causes depression, seizures, and Parkinson's disease symptoms such as tremors, shuffling gate, and flat affect (essentially, a blank stare). DOPA uses vitamin B6 for the reaction that creates dopamine, but one person's need for vitamin B6 for this reaction may be different than what someone else needs. Hence, there is what's called a "dosage response," meaning that the one amount of a nutrient may be insufficient for one person but enough for another person.

A combination of unique genetics and environmental factors affecting genetic expression causes a response or lack thereof in different people. This concept of *biochemical individuality* was observed in 1902 by Archibald E. Garrod, MD, a clinician in London, England, who wrote, "Individuals of a species do not conform to an absolutely rigid standard of metabolism but differ slightly in their chemistry as they do in their structure."[94] Nearly fifty-five years later, the eminent biochemist Roger J. Williams, PhD, published the book *Biochemical Individuality*, in which he observed, "Individuality in nutritional needs is the basis for the ... approach and for the belief that nutrition applied with due concern for individual genetic variations, which may be large, offers the solution to many baffling health problems."[14]

Bruce Ames, PhD, a UC Berkeley biochemist, has done pioneering work in this field.[22, 95-99] He determined that when two genes that produce the same enzyme for a given biochemical reaction differ between people, it commonly causes a decrease in the enzyme's ability to use the nutrient required for its reaction (e.g., a decrease in the ability of DOPA decarboxylase to use vitamin B6). This can be corrected by taking higher amounts of vitamin B6.

This field of study has been applied to *single nucleotide polymorphisms* (SNPs). An SNP is defined as a change in a gene that appears in more than

1% of the population.[100] Additionally, at least one-third of all SNPs decrease enzyme function.[98] This decreased function can, in many instances, be overcome by providing higher dosages of nutrients required by the enzyme. This approach has been proven effective repeatedly in studies of many different diseases.[12, 13, 98, 101] Readers are advised, however, that attempting to simply give themselves ever-higher dosages of nutrients without doing so under the guidance of a healthcare professional, who is an expert in nutritional medicine, carries risks of toxicity and is strongly discouraged by the authors.

A common example is the SNP for the methylene tetrahydrofolate reductase (MTHFR) enzyme. This enzyme is responsible for activating folic acid so that it can decrease homocysteine, a protein that increases your risk for cardiovascular disease, osteoporosis, cancer (colorectal, lung, cervical), and dementia.[102-108] Homocysteine causes these diseases through three distinct mechanisms: (1) it directly damages DNA by causing fragmentation of DNA in a way that mimics radiation exposure; (2) it directly damages the cells lining blood vessels (endothelial cells) and causes a decrease in oxygen and nutrient delivery to tissues such as the heart, brain, and bones; and (3) it directly decreases nitric oxide (NO) production, which causes narrowing of blood vessels, high blood pressure, and less oxygen and nutrient delivery to tissues.[109]

Variations in the genes that code for this enzyme decrease the activity of MTHFR by 30–65%. That is, the enzymes created by the different MTHFR SNPs require higher amounts of folic acid to function. These genetic changes occur in up to 50% of Caucasians, 47% of Koreans, 42% of Hispanics, 29% of Native Americans, 12% of African Americans, and 10% of Asian Indians. The deleterious effects of this genetic polymorphism can be overcome simply by providing higher dosages of folic acid.[100]

In addition to genetics, an enzyme's requirement for nutrients can increase due to hormones secreted during physical and psychological stress, lack of exercise, poor diet, and free-radical damage from the aging process. As people age, non-genetic factors (e.g., diet and lifestyle) play more important roles in the development of diseases than their genetics. In the vast majority of situations, genetics merely predisposes someone to a disease, but it is lifestyle and nutritional status that determine whether or not that disease will actually develop. The decreased ability to utilize nutrients can be overcome in many instances by giving higher dosages of the nutrient. This forces the reaction in the desired direction and helps reverse the harmful effects of aging and other stresses.

This fundamental concept has revolutionary implications for medicine. Medicine often looks at genetic alterations in their extreme forms (e.g., Down's Syndrome and Marfan's Syndrome). Subtle functional changes in biochemistry caused by genetic individuality, nutritional status, and lifestyle are much more common, and they often do not cause readily apparent physical or mental abnormalities. Instead, the changes in biochemical function are more inconspicuous, and the resultant diseases do not even appear until later in life.

In effect, the absolute amount of vitamin B6 people have in their bodies is not as important as whether they are functionally deficient in vitamin B6, or other vitamins, given their unique biochemistry. In the vast majority of people and diseases, genetics does not in and of itself create disease. A person's genetics merely predisposes them to diseases. Through sophisticated biochemical testing using a combination of urine and blood samples, truly personalized treatments for all sorts of diseases, including epilepsy, depression, chronic fatigue syndrome, fatigue, anxiety, and autism can be created. These and other conditions are discussed in subsequent chapters in this book.

CHAPTER FIVE

Mitochondria and Disease

Mitochondria are the powerhouses of our cells. Among other crucial functions, they generate energy as adenosine triphosphate (ATP) and heat. Current theory holds that mitochondria are the descendants of bacteria that colonized an ancient cell between one and three billion years ago.[110, 111] This allowed for the evolution of multicellular organisms such as humans. There are two areas in a cell that contain DNA—the nucleus and mitochondrion. The fact that mitochondria contain their own DNA is cited as evidence for the theory that mitochondria evolved from free-living bacteria.

Nuclear DNA is protected from free radical damage by proteins called histones. Mitochondrial DNA (mtDNA), however, lacks these proteins, and is therefore more susceptible to damage from free radicals. Mitochondrial injury by free radicals explains how mitochondria contribute to the creation and progression of diseases. The first mitochondrial disease was described in 1962, when a thirty-five-year-old woman experienced myopathy (muscle damage), excessive perspiration, heat intolerance (feeling hot when everyone else feels normal or cool), polydipsia (excessive thirst) with polyuria (excessive urination), and a metabolic rate 180% of normal.[112] The patient suffered from mitochondrial damage that resulted in the generation of heat without creating energy, which is why she felt hot. When samples of her muscle were taken and examined under a microscope, numerous enlarged mitochondria were seen. Just like muscles, when mitochondria have to work more, they get bigger. In her case, in order to produce enough energy to simply satisfy the minimum requirements of her body, her mitochondria had to work extremely hard.

Since then, mitochondrial dysfunction has been implicated in nearly all diseases (see table 4.1). These include acquired diseases such as diabetes, atherosclerosis, Parkinson's disease, Alzheimer's disease, sarcopenia (muscle wasting), and nonalcoholic steatohepatitis (enlarged, fatty liver not caused by alcoholism).

Table 4.1. Diseases associated with mitochondrial damage[99, 113-130]

Aging too rapidly
Alzheimer's disease
Anxiety disorders
Bipolar disorder
Cancer, including hepatitis-C virus-associated liver cancer
Cardiovascular disease, including atherosclerosis
Diabetes
Exercise intolerance
Fatigue, including chronic fatigue syndrome, fibromyalgia, and myofascial pain (pain arising from the connective tissue surrounding muscles)
Huntington's disease
Nonalcoholic steatohepatitis
Parkinson's disease
Sarcopenia
Schizophrenia

Symptoms of possible mitochondrial damage include weakness, muscle cramping and pain, atypical migraines, failure to gain weight, respiratory problems, absent or excessive sweating, atypical cerebral palsy, and more. However, since symptoms vary from case to case, age of onset, and rate of progression, mitochondrial dysfunction may not be diagnosed early on. Symptoms such as fatigue, muscle pain, shortness of breath, and abdominal pain can easily be mistaken for other diseases, such as chronic fatigue syndrome, fibromyalgia, or psychosomatic illness (symptoms caused by psychological conditions). Additionally, most doctors do not consider or test for mitochondrial dysfunction, which is best done through a series of blood and urine tests that can tell doctors where specific blocks in energy production pathways may exist.

Cellular energy requirements control the number of mitochondria per cell. A single cell can contain from two hundred to two thousand mitochondria.[131, 132] The largest numbers of mitochondria are found in the most metabolically active cells, such as skeletal muscle, cardiac muscle, liver, and brain. Mitochondria are found in every human cell except mature red blood cells.

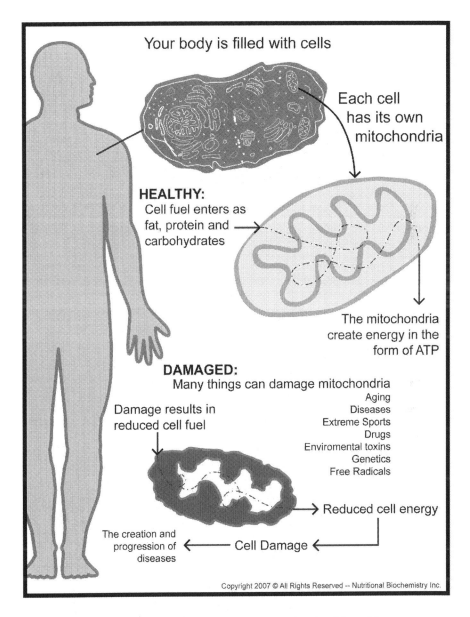

Figure 4.1. Protecting mitochondria is essential to health and longevity.

Mitochondria produce more than 90% of our cellular energy (ATP).[134] The biochemistry of energy production is quite complex, but basically energy is produced from the burning of sugars, fats, and proteins in cells (see figure 4.1). The efficient use of these fuels to produce energy requires various nutrients, such as magnesium, vitamin B1 (thiamin), vitamin B2 (riboflavin), vitamin B3 (niacin), L-carnitine, coenzyme Q10, alpha-lipoic acid, and others (see table 4.2).

Since the major reason for mitochondrial dysfunction is free-radical damage, it is not surprising that research has shown that antioxidant therapy helps repair mitochondrial dysfunction. Dietary supplements are not the only potential treatment strategy; diets rich in antioxidants can also help. However, since providing the wrong nutrients or excessive amounts of some nutrients, such as iron, can damage mitochondria further instead of repairing them, it's crucial that tests be run to determine exactly which nutrients a person needs. This testing is done with blood and urine samples, which provide clinicians with the information necessary to create customized treatment plans for patients.

Medication-Induced Mitochondrial Damage

Damage to mitochondria explains the side effects and dangers from pharmaceuticals. And when people take drug cocktails (multiple drugs simultaneously), they put themselves at even greater risk. The FDA does not require that drugs be tested for their ability to damage mitochondria, which may occur slowly over time.

The authors have concluded that people should assume all medications damage their mitochondria unless proven otherwise (see table 4.3). Simply stated, pharmaceuticals are poisons and every effort should be made to avoid taking them. The pharmaceutical industry and the FDA have substantial track records of selling drugs that later need to be recalled because of their harmful effects (e.g., Vioxx).

Table 4.2. Nutrients required for energy production[97, 133]

Vitamins	Minerals	Amino Acids
Biotin	Iron	L-carnitine
CoQ10	Magnesium	
Lipoic acid	Manganese	
Vitamin B1	Selenium	
Vitamin B2	Sulfur	
Vitamin B3	Zinc	
Vitamin B5	Copper	
Vitamin B6		
Vitamin C		
Vitamin E		

Table 4.3. Drugs documented to cause mitochondria damage[114, 135-141]

Drug class	Drugs
Alcoholism medications	Disulfiram (Antabuse)
Analgesic (for pain) and anti-inflammatory	aspirin, acetaminophen (Tylenol), diclofenac (Voltaren, Voltarol, Diclon, Dicloflex Difen and Cataflam), fenoprofen (Nalfon), indomethacin (Indocin, Indocid, Indochron E-R, Indocin-SR), naproxen (Aleve, Naprosyn)
Anesthetics	bupivacaine, lidocaine, propofol
Angina medications	perhexiline, amiodarone (Cordarone), diethylaminoethoxyhexesterol (DEAEH)
Antiarrhythmic (regulates heartbeat)	amiodarone (Cordarone)
Antibiotics	tetracycline, antimycin A
Antidepressants	amitriptyline (Lentizol), amoxapine (Asendis), citalopram (Cipramil), fluoxetine (Prozac, Symbyax, Sarafem, Fontex, Foxetin, Ladose, Fluctin, Prodep, Fludac, Oxetin, Seronil, Lovan)
Antipsychotics	chlorpromazine, fluphenazine, haloperidol, risperidone, quetiapine, clozapine, olanzapine
Anxiety medications	alprazolam (Xanax), diazepam (Valium, Diastat)
Barbiturates	amobarbital (Amytal), aprobarbital, butabarbital, butalbital (Fiorinal), hexobarbital (Sombulex), methylphenobarbital (Mebaral), pentobarbital (Nembutal), phenobarbital (Luminal), primidone, propofol, secobarbital (Seconal, Talbutal), thiobarbital
Cholesterol medications	statins: atorvastatin (Lipitor, Torvast), fluvastatin (Lescol), lovastatin (Mevacor, Altocor), pitavastatin (Livalo, Pitava), pravastatin (Pravachol, Selektine, Lipostat), rosuvastatin (Crestor), simvastatin (Zocor, Lipex)

	bile acidsholestyramine (Questran), clofibrate (Atromid-S), ciprofibrate (Modalim), colestipol (Colestid), colesevelam (Welchol)
Cancer (chemotherapy) medications	mitomycin C, profiromycin, adriamycin (also called doxorubicin and hydroxydaunorubicin and included in the following chemotherapeutic regimens: ABVD, CHOP and FAC)
Dementia	tacrine (Cognex), galantamine (Reminyl)
Diabetes medications	metformin (Fortamet, Glucophage, Glucophage XR, Riomet), troglitazone, rosiglitazone, buformin
HIV/AIDS medications	Atripla™, Combivir, Emtriva, Epivir (abacavir sulfate), Epzicom™, Hivid (ddc, zalcitabine), Retrovir (AZT, ZDV, zidovudine), Trizivir, Truvada, Videx (ddI, didanosine), Videx EC, Viread, Zerit (d4T, stavudine), Ziagen, Racivir
Epilepsy/Seizure medications	valproic acid (Depacon, Depakene, Depakene syrup, Depakote, Depakote ER, Depakote Sprinkle, Divalproex sodium)
Mood stabilizers	lithium
Parkinson's disease medications	tolcapone (Tasmar), entacapone (COMTan, also in the combination drug Stalevo)

In summary, mitochondria are the essential energy-producing part of our cells. Most diseases and medications damage mitochondria, which leads to a reduction in energy and the onset and progression of chronic, degenerative diseases. In essence, what is happening when mitochondria are damaged is that the body then begins to poison itself and cause its own deterioration, which can be tested for and corrected. Tests can identify actual decreases in the ability of mitochondria to produce energy, and they provide data that can be used to create customized treatment plans to repair, protect, and enhance mitochondrial function.

Chapter Six

Addictions

Many people have addictions that impact the quality of their life and can cause premature death. The causes and consequences of addictions are biochemical pathway abnormalities. An addiction is a repetitive behavior that, if stopped or impeded, creates symptoms of withdrawal such as anxiety, depression, irritability, tremors, nausea, and/or hallucinations. Examples of addictive substances or activities include alcohol, drugs (narcotics, methamphetamines, marijuana), work, sex, extreme danger, exercise, and foods (e.g., sugar). Not all types of drinking behaviors would be classified as an addiction, but the compulsion to take a drink, which the person rationalizes as a necessity, signifies an addiction.

Addictions can be very subtle and at the same time very lethal. For example, going to work is a normal behavior. The need to work compulsively, meaning that someone's entire life revolves around work, is a symptom of a workaholic. And what makes this definition more complicated is that society can rationalize this behavior as very positive because the person is making money, earning a living for his or her family, and enhancing his or her self-esteem. But the key element here is that if the person takes a few days off of work, they may become restless, irritable, anxious, and experience insomnia, headaches, and depression.

Dopamine, a brain chemical linked to pleasure and elation, also has a dark side—a link to addiction. Nora Volkow of Brookhaven National Laboratory, a world leader in addiction research, has explored this link in detail. Volkow has shown that addicts have fewer-than-average dopamine receptors in their brains, so that weaker dopamine signals are sent between cells, and life naturally has less joy. Addicts thus are encouraged to derive pleasure from dopamine-stimulant drugs, such as alcohol, cocaine, and nicotine. This cycle was first identified in 1990 when Volkow and coworkers showed that cocaine addiction inhibits the dopamine signaling system. Using positron-emission tomography, they determined the critical biochemical changes and where they occur in the brain in response to addictive drugs. These studies demonstrated that addictions are associated with high levels of dopamine in a pleasure center in the brain. The decreased ability to utilize dopamine means people need more to feel the pleasure other people experience with lower dopamine levels. The findings have been proven again and again in studies of addictions to drugs and food/overeating.[142-144]

The biochemistry of food addiction follows a path that is initiated when refined carbohydrates flood the brain with dopamine, serotonin, and epinephrine. As the brain becomes flooded with these neurotransmitters, a feeling of well-being results and craving is stimulated. This simultaneously creates a deficiency in the brain because carbohydrates block the recycling of neurotransmitters (e.g., dopamine, serotonin, epinephrine). Thus the brain becomes depleted of needed neurotransmitters. This "feast followed by famine" of brain chemicals upsets the hypothalamus, which is the brain's center for emotions and survival. Therefore, mood and cravings go out of control.

The result is that one is walking around "drunk" on refined carbohydrates. During this process, an insufficiency of neurotransmitters leaves receptor sites unfilled. This puts the brain in a condition of imbalance, resulting in distress and depression as well as cravings. It takes increasingly larger and more frequent amounts of carbohydrates to bring the brain back into balance. Over long periods of time, food addicts are unable to get back to baseline. To feel better, they continue to eat that which makes them feel worse. Morgan Spurlock, in the excellent documentary titled *Super Size Me*, demonstrated this situation. In this film, Mr. Spurlock dedicated himself to eating only McDonald's food for a month. He comments in the documentary how at first the food left him feeling terrible, but as his body became accustomed to it, if he didn't eat it he felt terrible. His biochemistry had changed and he became addicted, even though the food itself was poisoning his body. During the month, doctors tracked his health and ran tests that showed the food was causing significant damage to his body.

In the traditional approach, the only option for recovering from food addictions is to abstain from those chemicals that trigger the addictive response. In order to accomplish recovery, food addicts learn to be scrupulous about identifying all the substances that induce active addiction at the physical level. However, a more fundamental and comprehensive approach to combating addiction also tests for biochemical-pathway abnormalities and provides sufficient amounts of the appropriate nutrients to correct biochemical imbalances. The fact that people may be predisposed to addiction due to reduced dopamine receptors may be compensated for by stimulating the body to naturally produce more dopamine by providing higher dosages of the nutrients, such as vitamin B6, needed for its production. Addiction to sugar may caused by a decreased ability to control proper blood sugar levels due to low chromium, vanadium, carnitine, and essential amino acids. Additionally, serotonin and norepinephrine pathways involved in addictive behavior can be tested for and nutritionally enhanced. The tests for these pathways and their nutrients consist of urinary-organic acids, plasma-amino acids, and intracellular minerals.[63] In essence, cravings are highly determined by physiology and biochemistry. Using this nutritional medicine approach, cravings for addictive substances may be decreased quicker, thus allowing people to more easily beat their addictions.

CHAPTER SEVEN

Osteoporosis

Osteoporosis is caused by bone loss that results in an increased risk for fractures. There are two types of osteoporosis. Type I is most commonly associated with postmenopausal women, fifty to seventy years old, in which estrogen deficiency is the assumed cause. Here fractures of the wrist and spine are common. Type II osteoporosis is associated with aging and assumed to be from a reduction in calcium absorption. This affects an older group (over seventy years of age) and results more often in hip fractures. Osteoporosis may also occur due to calcium deficiency, physical inactivity, elevated cortisol, hyperthyroidism, and steroid medications (e.g., Prednisone).

Osteoporosis is a major epidemic in industrialized nations. In the United States, 1.2 million fractures occur each year, mostly in women, as a direct result of osteoporosis. Figures from the National Osteoporosis Foundation indicate that about forty-four million Americans are at risk for the disease by virtue of having low bone mineral densities. Presently ten million adults have osteoporosis. Nationally, the direct expenditure on treating the 1.5 million fractures that occur each year associated with osteoporosis is approximately forty-seven million dollars a day. Almost a quarter of the patients over fifty years of age die within one year of their hip fracture.[145]

Bone remodeling is the function of the activity of two different cell lines. Osteoblasts, which build bone, respond to changes in the activity of osteoclasts, which break down bone. Many hormones, growth factors, and cytokines (signaling molecules produced by cells) play a regulatory role in maintaining bone by their effects on these two cell lines. Estrogen in particular is responsible for suppressing osteoclast activity and thereby preventing bone loss, which explains why the rate of bone degeneration increases in women after menopause. However, in acute ovarian estrogen deficiency, which occurs in surgical or natural menopause, the rate of bone resorption due to increased osteoclast activity exceeds the rate at which osteoblasts are capable of forming new bone.

The net result is depletion of calcium, collagen, and protein from bone, and increased porosity and risk for fracture. Estrogen receptors ERα and ERβ are both found on human osteoblasts, although the expression of these subtypes varies considerably during cell maturation. The greatly increased expression of ERβ during bone mineralization is particularly pertinent to the potential hormonal effects of phytoestrogens (estrogens in plants) because compounds such as genistein from soy show a much higher affinity for ERβ than for ERα. This is the underlying mechanism by which soy phytoestrogens have been shown in clinical trials to reduce the rate of bone breakdown and contribute to increasing bone mineralization.[145]

There are additional risk factors for osteoporosis, such as a sedentary lifestyle, depression, chronic stress, and nutrient deficiencies (see table 6.1). Weight-bearing exercise is one of the most common suggestions for decreasing osteoporosis risk and slowing its progression. Muscles attach to bones, and when people lift weights it puts a strain on those attachments. This stimulates osteoblasts to create more bone. Depression and chronic stress both entail activation of the sympathetic nervous system. The sympathetic nervous system releases epinephrine, which causes a breakdown in bone matrix. Nutrient deficiencies, aside from decreasing the raw materials necessary for bone creation, can cause depression and stress.

Table 6.1. Lifestyle and metabolic factors affecting bone health

Increases Bone Health	Decreases Bone Health
Weight-bearing exercise	Sedentary lifestyle
Stress reduction	Smoking
Vitamin D	Alcohol
Minerals (calcium, boron, zinc, magnesium)	Low vitamin D status
Amino acids	Low minerals (boron, calcium, chromium, copper, magnesium, vanadium, zinc)
Soy phytoestrogens	Increased urinary-bone-specific collagen
	Depression
	Psychological stress
	Elevated homocysteine

Currently, several technologies can measure bone-mineral density. The most commonly used method is called dual-energy X-ray absorptiometry (DEXA). This technique can measure the bone density of the hip and spine within a few percentages. DEXA has largely taken the place of dual-photon absorptiometry because the latter may fail to distinguish true bone mineral from osteophytes (bone spurs) in the lumbar spine. Bone-density measurements at the distal radius (in the wrist) or calcaneus (in the foot) are more convenient and less expensive than DEXA. However, while these tests may help predict fracture risk, bone density at distal sites does not necessarily correlate with bone density of the hip and spine, where most of the medically significant fractures occur. Even hip and spine measurements provide only a rough estimate of fracture risk. For example, some individuals with very "dense" bones develop osteoporotic fractures, whereas many people with frank bone loss never suffer a fracture. Evidently, bone-mineral content is only one factor; the quality of the bone crystal (which cannot be readily measured) also appears to be important.

Bone is a tissue, and, like all tissues, it's a complex mixture of elements. Minerals, such as calcium, magnesium, and boron give bone its hardness, while collagen (connective tissue) supplies its flexibility. The collagen provides the underlying structure onto which the minerals attach. Therefore, if the collagen is being destroyed, the minerals are not held in place as well.

To get a fuller picture of bone health and osteoporosis risk, additional testing beyond a simple bone-density scan is necessary. Available urine and blood measure various markers of bone resorption (such as urinary N-telopeptide crosslinks and pyridinoline) and bone formation (such as serum osteocalcin and bone-specific alkaline phosphatase). Studies have shown that these markers can predict changes in bone density as detected by subsequent DEXA tests (see table 6.2).

One specific marker found in urine is bone-specific deoxypyridinoline (DPD).[146] Detection of this protein signifies the breakdown of bone collagen, and elevated urinary DPD indicates increased osteoporosis risk and progression. One benefit of testing urinary DPD is that it can be retested more frequently than a DEXA scan, which allows doctors to more closely monitor and adjust treatments. The precision of DEXA is only about 3%, whereas bone density may change by less than 3% per year.[147] Repeating the test too soon may therefore provide nothing more than expensive and unreliable data points. Doctors usually advise patients to wait eighteen to twenty-four months before repeating their DEXA test, which is a crude way to monitor the progression of osteoporosis. In contrast, urinary DPD can be retested every four to six weeks and decreased. Research has shown that specific nutritional protocols can increase bone mineral density by 1.5% to 5% on repeat DEXA scans.[148-155]

Table 6.2. Laboratory variables tested and their effects on bone health

Analyte	Effects on bone health
Homocysteine	Can damage blood vessels and decrease nutrient delivery to bone
Bone-specific collagen	Specific marker for bone-collagen destruction
Amino acids	Low amino acids can indicate decreased digestion.
Magnesium	Low magnesium may result in decreased bone mineralization.
Vitamin D	Low vitamin D decreases calcium absorption in the small intestines and is associated with increased risk of falls and osteoporotic fractures.
Zinc	Required for bone mineralization
Copper	Required for bone mineralization
Chromium	Required for bone mineralization
Vanadium	Required for bone mineralization
IgG 1&4 food antigens	Can cause decreased digestion and absorption of nutrients required for bone health

Although testing for osteoporosis can provide a rough estimate of fracture risk, no single test or combination of tests is 100% reliable. Considering the epidemic nature of osteoporosis, everyone should consider a prevention program, including a diet of whole foods, supplementation with calcium and other micronutrients, regular weight-bearing exercise, and abstaining from cigarettes and excessive amounts of caffeine and alcohol. Other nutritional factors and variables, such as vitamin D and homocysteine, should also be tested. Clinical trials have shown that increasing vitamin D levels decreases the risk of falls and fractures in people with osteoporosis.[156, 157]

Additionally, some medications increase one's risk for osteoporosis.[76] These include acid-blocking medications such Protonix, Tagamet, Pepcid, Axid, Zantac, Prevacid, Prilosec, Aciphex, and Nexium. People may be able to discontinue these medications, but they should first have proper testing conducted to determine the best way to treat any underlying dysfunction so these medications are no longer necessary.

Although osteoporosis is an epidemic and causes premature death, in many cases it is preventable and treatable using a combination of improved diet, healthy lifestyle, and nutritional medicine. A proactive approach to bone health is the best way to ensure people are doing everything possible to stay healthy as long as they can.

Chapter Eight

Fatigue and Depression

Fatigue and depression are related. One cardinal sign of depression is that a person sleeps longer, and a consequence of fatigue is depression. Additionally, chronic pain also causes sleep disturbances, fatigue, and depression. Fatigue and depression are combined into one chapter because of the similarities in testing results and in treatment strategies.

The essential concept in this chapter is that specific biochemical pathways control and influence mood and energy levels. As mentioned in chapter five, these pathways require B-complex vitamins, minerals such as magnesium and manganese, amino acids such as L-carnitine, and other nutrients such as alpha lipoic acid. If a person is functionally deficient in nutrients required for these pathways, energy production can decrease and fatigue ensues. The link between essential amino acids (those amino acids that can only be obtained from food since the body cannot manufacture them) has been known for more than fifty years. In the early 1950s, researchers identified essential amino acids and discovered that low levels of any one of them (e.g., phenylalanine, leucine, isoleucine, valine, tryptophan, etc.) caused a "failure in appetite, a sensation of extreme fatigue, and an increase in nervous irritability."[158-161] Pathways effecting mood and energy can be tested using a combination of urinary-organic acids, plasma-amino acids, and intracellular minerals.

While the effects of specific nutrients and pathways on fatigue and depression are well documented (see figures 7.1a and 7.1b), conventional medicine ignores them. Instead of providing customized treatments based on a person's specific biochemical needs, conventional medicine adopts a one-size-fits-all approach to depression by prescribing antidepressant medications. These medications fall into two classes—selective serotonin reuptake inhibitors (SSRI) and selective serotonin and norepinephrine reuptake inhibitors (SNRI). Examples of SSRI medications include Zoloft, Lexapro, Celexa, and Prozac, and an example of a SNRI medication is Welbutrin.

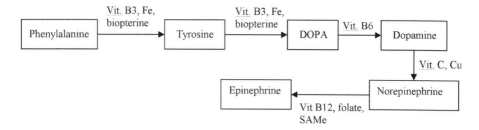

Figure 7.1a. Low dopamine and epinephrine can cause fatigue and depression. The SNRI medications work on this pathway to artificially increase dopamine and epinephrine, but people can be deficient in phenylalanine, tyrosine, or vitamins and minerals required for dopamine and epinephrine production. When testing reveals the exact deficiency, nutrients can be supplied to aid the body in producing its own dopamine and serotonin naturally, without medications. Moreover, the natural approach is nearly devoid of any risk for side effects while the SNRI medications carry significant risk of serious side effects.

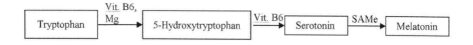

Figure 7.1b. The essential amino acid L-tryptophan and vitamin B6 are required for the production of serotonin and melatonin. Serotonin helps control mood and melatonin helps people sleep. The SSRI and SNRI medications increase serotonin by decreasing its breakdown instead of providing the raw materials for effective serotonin production. Abbreviations: Mg = Magnesium; SAMe = S-adenosyl methionine; Vit. B6 = Vitamin B6.

Many people turn to stimulants and short-term solutions to lift their spirits and energy such as alcohol, sugar, caffeine, cocaine, methamphetamines, and Ritalin. These substances provide brief relief from the symptoms of fatigue and depression, but in effect they make the underlying causes of the problems worse. For example, sugar directly stimulates a release of serotonin in the central nervous system, thereby lifting mood, and it also provides fuel for energy production. The problem is that eating sugar also stimulates insulin release because insulin's job is to help move sugar from the blood stream and into cells that use the sugar for energy. But when this happens, blood sugar drops and the person becomes hypoglycemic (having low blood sugar), which manifests itself in the symptoms of irritability, restlessness, insomnia, fatigue, and depression.[162] The paradox here is that even though people feel fatigued, they also feel restless and may have insomnia because of the subsequent low serotonin and melatonin.

There is another irony here. Most people who feel depressed and tired often drink alcohol to sleep, but within a few hours they wake up with increased irritability, restlessness, and insomnia, which can become intractable since the more they feel these symptoms the more they want to drink in order to eliminate them. The alcohol itself is a central nervous system depressant, but it's also just fermented sugar, and alcoholic beverages therefore contain high amounts of carbohydrates. The rebound effect on mood and energy is explained by the same mechanisms as sugar itself. When blood sugar drops too low during sleep, it stimulates the release of cortisol and epinephrine. These hormones cause the release of stored sugars in the body to raise blood sugar, but they also wake people up. The more someone drinks and the more someone eats sugar to lift their mood, the more their problems are compounded because of the resultant hypoglycemia.

An additional factor is that as people eat more sugar and drink more alcohol, the consumption of nutrient-dense foods containing essential vitamins, minerals, and amino acids decreases. So if the cause for depression and fatigue is a deficiency in the compounds required for healthy neurotransmitter production, masking the symptoms by consuming sugar, alcohol, and other substances that provide a short-term boost in mood and energy actually worsens the depression and fatigue. This becomes a vicious cycle that people have great difficulty breaking out of because the withdrawal effects can be more severe than the addiction. For example, delirium tremens results from alcohol withdrawal when one is addicted to alcohol. Symptoms of delirium tremens consist of visual and auditory hallucinations, hyperthermia, tremors, insomnia, fecal and urinary incontinence, and depression.[163, 164] The regulatory mechanisms that keep these systems in balance are completely derailed. This is a medical emergency.

Caffeine is one of the most-abused drugs in this country. Caffeine provides a quick boost in energy but drains energy when used in excess. Caffeine is a diuretic, which means that it increases urine production. In the process, it decreases water-soluble vitamins, such as the B vitamins that are required for producing energy and regulating mood. Caffeine addiction can also cause fatal irregularities in heartbeat called atrial fibrillation, which is experienced as a fluttering in the chest.[165]

The authors are very concerned about the amount of caffeine that young people consume. An eight-ounce can of Red Bull, an energy drink, contains eighty milligrams of caffeine, a twelve-ounce can of Jolt contains seventy-one milligrams, and Mountain Dew contains fifty-five milligrams. In contrast, depending on the brewing method, one eight-ounce cup of coffee delivers eighty to one hundred seventy five milligrams of caffeine. On the low end, instant coffee contains sixty-five to one hundred milligrams of caffeine, and on the high end, drip coffee delivers one hundred fifteen to one hundred seventy five milligrams of caffeine per eight-ounce cup. These nutrient depletions can cause addictions, chronic and degenerative diseases (e.g., osteoporosis, osteoarthritis, heart disease), and decreased cognitive function.

Again, while caffeine delivers a quick boost like alcohol, it depletes the very source of cellular energy production. What makes coffee shops so popular is that they are vehicles for delivering and feeding caffeine addictions to millions of people everyday. When someone abruptly stops drinking coffee, they can experience rebound effects such as fatigue, irritability, constipation, and headaches.

Biochemical testing can detect specific deficiencies in pathways that control mood and energy (see table 7.1). This approach is much more sophisticated than simply providing medications to treat the symptoms, and it allows skilled clinicians to correct the underlying biochemical causes.

Table 7.1. Laboratory analytes in the evaluation of fatigue and depression[63, 166, 167]

Analytes	Results	Comments
5-hydroxyindoleacetate	Low	Indicates low serotonin, which can cause depression and fatigue
Adipate, suberate, ethyl-malonate	High	Functional deficiency in L-carnitine
Aluminum, arsenic, cadmium, lead, mercury	High	Mitochondrial damage and decreased energy production
Ethanolamine	High	Depression
Ferritin	Low	Ferritin is the storage form of iron and is *the* most sensitive indicator for iron-deficiency anemia. Low iron causes fatigue, depression, and mitochondrial damage.

Gamma-amino-butyric acid (GABA)	Low	Depression
Glutamate	Low	Depression and fatigue
Glutamine	High	Fatigue
Glycine	Low	Anemia and depression
Homovanillate (HVA)	Low	Indicates low dopamine, which can cause fatigue, depression and Parkinson's symptoms.
Magnesium	Low	Low magnesium can result in decreased energy production.
Methylmalonic acid	High	Indicates low vitamin B12, which can cause fatigue and depression
Omega-3 fatty acids	Low	Can cause depression
Phenylalanine	Low/ High	An essential amino acid; low amounts mean inadequate dietary intake. Elevated amounts mean decreased conversion to tyrosine for thyroid hormone production. Both situations can result in depression and fatigue.
Serine-to-glycine ratio	High	Depression
Taurine	High	Depression
Tryptophan	Low	Results in low serotonin and melatonin production, causing depression and insomnia, respectively
Tyrosine	Low	Low tyrosine can result in low thyroid hormone production and resultant fatigue and depression.
Vanilmandelate (VMA)	Low	Indicates low epinephrine production, which can cause fatigue and depression

Xanthurenate	High	Low vitamin B6, which decreases the conversion of tryptophan to serotonin, and the conversion of DOPA to dopamine, which can also cause depression
α-Ketoisovalerate, α-Ketoisocaproate, α-Keto-β-methylvalerate	High	Functional deficiencies in vitamins B1, B2, B3, B5, and lipoic acid

CHAPTER NINE

Exercise Stamina and Strength

Exercise is an excellent way to improve one's health and prevent many chronic, degenerative diseases such as heart disease, diabetes, and cancer. However, like everything, moderation is the key. Moderate exercise can strengthen muscles, improve circulation and immune function, and decrease stress. For example, a thirty-minute workout three to five days weekly is considered beneficial.

But extreme sports can be detrimental. Extreme sports include running marathons, decathlons, the Iron Man race, mountain climbing, and long-distance bike racing. All these place extreme demands on the body's biochemical pathways. During exercise, there is increased demand for energy production. The generation of cellular energy involves the metabolism of carbohydrates, fats, and proteins. The body first utilizes carbohydrates then, as the energy demand continues, the body begins breaking down fats and will finally resort to using proteins when the supply of fats is not sufficient to meet demands.

The problem is that muscles store the proteins used for energy. Therefore, when the body needs proteins to create energy during extreme sports, it actually begins breaking down muscle. A consequence is that in trying to do something healthy and build strength and endurance, people are actually causing the opposite—they become weaker and have less endurance over time. These activities are not sustainable in the long run, and that's why young people dominate these sports.

In addition to cannibalizing muscle to sustain energy, extreme sports also disrupt the body's antioxidant system.[168] While moderate exercise increases antioxidants, extreme exercise depletes antioxidants and increases free-radical damage to cells.[168] This is because producing energy also creates free radicals, as explained in chapter five. The end result is mitochondrial damage and a decreased ability to produce more energy.

The stress from extreme sports also depletes the water-soluble vitamins (B-complex vitamins and vitamin C). Every person who participates in extreme sports can tell you stories of severe muscle burning. In some cases they describe it as "hitting the wall." What happens is that lactic acid builds up and causes the burning. This is referred to technically as *lactic acidosis*. People may be under the impression that they need to be mentally tough and work through this burning sensation when in fact what they're doing is trying to override an important message from the body. The burning experienced during exercise is the body's way of saying that it's in serious trouble since carbohydrates can no longer effectively flow down their pathway to generate energy. The block in the pathway is a result of nutrient depletions due to the stress placed on the body.

Many people believe that the sudden death that can occur in marathon runners is a result of cardiac arrhythmia. But it is the authors' belief that what in fact happens in many of the health clubs is that the individual experiences immediate exertion onset bronchospasms due to depletion of the nutrients necessary for the production of epinephrine required for breathing. This situation is a result of chronically low nutrient levels and mitochondrial damage that appear when an added physical stress, such as exercise, is placed on the body, and the demands for energy production and epinephrine are greatly increased. The body simply does not have the ability to keep up with the demand placed on it.

Exercise stamina and muscle strength can also decrease as people age even without participating in extreme sports. This is due to nutrient depletions such as decreased amino acids, vitamins, and minerals. When biochemical testing is performed on athletes who engage in extreme sports and on the elderly who are experiencing muscle burning and muscle weakness, the test results can be strikingly similar (table 8.1).

Table 8.1. Symptoms and underlying biochemical dysfunctions in exercise stamina and strength

Symptoms	Underlying biochemical dysfunctions
Muscle burning	Lactic-acid buildup from mitochondrial damage and nutrient deficiencies
Weakness	Deficiencies in the essential amino acids leucine, isoleucine, and valine, and also of vitamin B6 required for their utilization

Decreased stamina	Lactic-acid buildup from mitochondrial damage and nutrient deficiencies—deficiencies in the essential amino acids leucine, isoleucine, and valine.
Shortness of breath	Decreased epinephrine production.
Degenerative joint disease	Decreased amino acids proline and glycine; increased free-radical damage; decreased zinc.

While exercise can be beneficial and is an important part of a healthy lifestyle, it is problematic that more and more people in the United States are going to extremes—either over-exercising or not exercising enough. It's no accident that obesity and anorexia are both at epidemic proportions in the United States. Extreme sports have become a national addiction for many sociological reasons that are beyond the scope of this book. But what is important is to undergo a thorough biochemical evaluation that will analyze the four hundred plus analytes that are essential for proper biochemical function. This approach can help identify which pathways are already deficient or will become deficient.

On a more optimistic note, there are nutrients and compounds that can prevent the problems that develop during exercise. However, these nutrients must be in the proper proportions and of high quality to provide the necessary benefits that people need to promote and maintain their health. It's important to note that for many reasons, these are not the products you will find in the drugstores or stores advertising "ripped physiques" and muscle-building formulas.

CHAPTER TEN

Memory Loss
and Dementia

Many people, including the authors, want to maintain their memory and vitality for as long as possible. Memory loss can occur normally as people age or abnormally from many different situations. Head trauma during a car accident or a sporting incident can create what is called *retrograde amnesia*. That is, people know what happened before and after the accident, but they do not remember the accident itself. Metabolic disturbances that decrease memory can also occur, including loss of memory by alcoholics due to a vitamin B1 deficiency, called Wernicke's encephalopathy. Alcoholics and elderly people who experience memory loss may compensate by inventing information to fill the gaps in their memories, such as dates, places, and people. The ability to accurately state the day's date, the place in which the person is, and who is with the person is one way that doctors screen for memory loss. The act of creating information is called *confabulation*.

Dementia differs from memory loss in its severity and ability to incapacitate the mind and body. Dementia is the loss of mental functions—such as thinking, memory, and reasoning—that is severe enough to interfere with a person's daily functioning. Dementia is not a disease itself, but rather a group of symptoms that might accompany certain diseases or conditions. Symptoms also might include changes in personality, mood, and behavior.

Dementia affects only 1% of people aged sixty to sixty-four but 30–50% of those older than eighty-five years. In the United States, about four to five million people are affected. Dementia is the leading cause of institutionalization among the elderly, and about 60–80% of all elderly nursing home residents have dementia.[169] Dementia is irreversible when caused by disease or injury, but it might be reversible when caused by drugs, alcohol, hormone, vitamin imbalances or depression.

Dementia develops when the parts of the brain that are involved with learning, memory, decision-making, and language are affected by any one of various infections or diseases. The most common cause of dementia is Alzheimer's disease, but there are as many as fifty other known causes. Most of these causes are very rare.

Some of the disorders that cause memory loss and dementia might be reversible, although, unfortunately, most types of dementia do not respond to treatment. Therefore, it is very important to evaluate dementia symptoms comprehensively, so as not to miss potentially treatable conditions. The frequency of "treatable" causes of dementia is believed to be about 20%.

Treatable causes of memory loss and dementia are reversible disorders that can be cured completely or partially by addressing the underlying problem. Because some types of dementia are treatable, it is important not to assume that a person who is showing symptoms of dementia is suffering from Alzheimer's disease or another incurable disease (table 9.1).

Table 9.1. Treatable and non-treatable causes of memory loss and dementia

Treatable	Non-treatable
Chronic drug abuse	Alzheimer's disease
Tumors that can be removed	Multi-infarct dementia
Subdural hematoma (accumulation of blood beneath the outer covering of the brain that results from a broken blood vessel, usually as a result of a head injury)	Dementias associated with Parkinson's disease and similar disorders
Normal pressure hydrocephalus (enlarged regions of the brain)	AIDS dementia complex (currently considered non-treatable, but may be treatable since AIDS medications are mitochondrial poisons, which may lead to dementia)
Metabolic disorders, such as a vitamin B12 deficiency	Creutzfeldt-Jakob disease (CJD), a quickly progressing and fatal disease that is characterized by dementia and myoclonus (muscle twitching and spasms), popularly known as mad cow disease

Hypothyroidism (low levels of thyroid hormone)	
Hypoglycemia (low blood sugar)	

The biochemical aspects of memory loss have been extensively studied. While many questions remain unanswered, much is already known that can provide relief to millions. Acetylcholine, a neurotransmitter in the brain and rest of the body, is needed for memory formation and recall. Rivastigmine, an alkaloid derived from a plant, is an example of an FDA-approved pharmacological agent that preserves acetylcholine. It is in a class of medications called *cholinesterase inhibitors*. These drugs decrease the breakdown of acetylcholine, thereby increasing the amount of acetylcholine that remains. Acetylcholine is essential for memory and muscle control. Research has shows that rivastigmine also increases mitochondrial energy production.[170] Animal studies using huperzine A, a naturally occurring plant extract derived from the plant *Huperzia serrata*, showed that it is as effective at increasing acetylcholine levels in the brain as the medication donepezil and rivastigmine.[171] Clinical trials in China, where the plant originates, have shown significant increases in memory when people with memory loss and dementia took huperzine A.[172]

As the name implies, acetylcholine is comprised of two components—acetyl and choline. The acetyl portion comes from vitamin B5 and choline can be synthesized in the body from any of the amino acids threonine, glycine, and serine. The synthesis of choline from these precursors requires the mineral manganese and the vitamins folic acid and B6.[63]

Although choline is not classified as a vitamin, it is an essential nutrient. Despite the fact that choline can be synthesized in small amounts in people, it must be consumed in the diet to maintain good health. Choline is found in high quantities in beef liver, wheat germ, eggs, and salmon (see table 9.2).

Table 9.2. Dietary sources of choline[173]

Food	Serving	Total Choline (mg)
Beef liver, pan fried	3 ounces*	355
Wheat germ, toasted	1 cup	172
Egg	1 large	126
Atlantic cod, cooked	3 ounces	71
Beef, trim cut, cooked	3 ounces	66

Brussels sprouts, cooked	1 cup	63
Broccoli, cooked	1 cup, chopped	62
Salmon	3 ounces	56
Shrimp, canned	3 ounces	49
Peanut butter, smooth	2 tablespoons	20
Milk chocolate	1.5-ounce bar	20

*A three-ounce serving of meat or fish is about the size of a deck of cards.

Consuming vitamin B5 and choline may stimulate the production of acetylcholine, thereby increasing the production of molecules essential for memory. Promoting mitochondrial function in the brain can also improve memory. Dr. Bruce Ames of UC Berkeley has conducted research in mice showing that providing adequate amount of acetyl-L-carnitine and other nutrients improve memory and cognitive function. Carnitine is an amino acid that stimulates the breakdown of fats for cellular energy. Two-thirds of the brain is fat, and providing nutrients that stimulate the pathways for energy production in the brain can help increase memory and cognitive function, which are energy-intensive processes.

Many people are also at increased risk for memory loss and dementia because of elevated homocysteine and free-radical damage to the hippocampus, a region of the brain that controls short-term memory. Homocysteine is an amino acid derived from methionine. Homocysteine causes damage to blood vessels and decreased blood flow to tissues such as the brain. This can cause low oxygen and nutrient delivery to the brain. The results are an increase in free-radical damage to the hippocampus and other regions of the brain, damaged mitochondria, and decreased energy production in the central nervous system.

Chronic stress also increases the risk of memory loss due to free-radical damage to the hippocampus. Psychological and physiological stresses cause release of cortisol, which has many

---

Effects of chronic stress on the brain

The hippocampus has high levels of cortisol receptors, and chronic stress impairs hippocampal function leading to:

- **Neuronal atrophy and destruction**
- **Decreased short term memory**
- **Decreased contextual memory**
- **Poor regulation of endocrine response to stress**

Reference: McEwen BS. Protective and damaging effects of stress mediators. *New England Journal of Medicine.* 1998; 338(3):171–179.

effects on the body, including the alteration of blood flow in the brain and damage to mitochondria. Cortisol is part of the fight or flight system in the body. During the fight or flight response, cortisol decreases blood flow to the medial temporal lobe[174] and sugar utilization for energy production in the hippocampus.[175] The hippocampus is considered part of the medial temporal lobe, which controls memory.[176] Research shows that people with chronic cortisol elevations have a nearly 20% destruction of their hippocampus and also destruction of the frontal lobe.[177] Protecting the brain with a balanced lifestyle that includes relaxation, healthy eating, and dietary supplements to protect and restore brain function are crucial to preventing and improving memory loss and dementia.

Testing can evaluate the biochemical risk factors for memory loss and dementia. Risk factors include elevated homocysteine, lipid peroxides (free-radical damage to cell membranes), 8-hydroxy-2-deoxyguanosine (free-radical damage to DNA) and glutamate (neurotoxin), and decreased vitamin B12 and folic acid (see table 9.3.)

Table 9.3. Essential analytes evaluating risk for memory loss and dementia[63, 178-180]

Analytes	Comments
Homocysteine	Increases vascular damage and decreased nutrients and oxygen to the brain
Lipid peroxides	Indicates free radical damage to cell membranes
Glutamate	An excitatory neurotransmitter in the brain and a toxin to brain cells
Alpha-ketoisocaproate	High levels indicate low B-vitamins
Alpha-keto-beta-methylvalarate	High levels indicate low B-vitamins
Xanthurenate	High levels indicate low vitamin B6
Beta-hydroxyisovalerate	High levels indicate low B-vitamins
Essential amino acids	Required for hormones and brain function
Methylmalonic acid	Indicates vitamin B12 deficiency
Formiminoglutamate	Indicates folic acid deficiency

Toxic metals (aluminum, arsenic, cadmium, lead, mercury)	Toxic to mitochondria and brain cells

In conclusion, the lifestyle and predisposing biochemical factors that contribute to the development of memory loss and dementia are well documented. Preserving brain function through testing and aggressive dietary and lifestyle modifications provides the greatest hope for decreasing the epidemic of memory loss and dementia. Studies show that nutritional interventions can be effective in increasing memory and slowing the progression of dementia. Again, it is crucial to test for biochemical pathways and optimal nutritional status to ensure the body has what it needs to function optimally. What appear to be serious and inevitable problems, like memory loss and dementia, are in fact merely well-documented dysfunctions in biochemical pathways, which may be corrected. The most comprehensive biochemical test that evaluates four hundred different analytes is indispensable.

CHAPTER ELEVEN

Overweight and Obese

Overweight and obese are two terms for a spectrum of dangerous metabolic conditions that result in increased risk of diabetes, heart disease, cancer, degenerative joint disease, and premature death. Obesity in the United States has increased at "an epidemic rate" over the last twenty years. The percentage of U.S. adults classified as overweight increased from 56% in 1994 to 65% in 2002, and obesity increased from 23% to 30% during this same time period. Approximately 16% of children and adolescents six to nineteen years old were overweight in 2002.[181-183]

Obesity is defined as an excessively high amount of body fat relative to muscle mass. There are many ways to measure obesity, including skin fold measurements, waist-to-hip circumference ratio, ultrasound, computed tomography, magnetic resonance imaging, and more. One of the most commonly used measurements, however, is the body mass index (BMI), which calculates the ratio of weight-to-height, using the equation weight in centimeters divided by height in meters squared (wt/ht^2). The World Health Organization (WHO) defines overweight as a BMI of 25-29.9, while a BMI of ≥ 30 is considered obese. Obesity is further divided into grades I, II, and III. Grade I obesity is a BMI of 30-34.9, Grade II obesity is a BMI of 35-39.4, and Grade III obesity is a BMI ≥ 40.

A wide range of health consequences exist for those who are overweight, including increased risk of diabetes; cardiovascular disease, including hypertension, coronary heart disease, angina pectoris, congestive heart failure, and stroke; gallstones; sleep apnea; some cancers, such as endometrial, breast, prostate, and colon cancers; complications of pregnancy; incontinence; and depression. Obesity can lead to early death.

Many people trying to lose weight experience extreme difficulty because of alterations in their biochemistry. There are three crucial reasons for this. One is that obese people consume very calorie-rich, nutrient poor foods. For example, processed foods, such as potato chips, are high in carbohydrates, trans fats, and salt, and they are essentially devoid of vitamins and minerals. A McDonald's Big Mac (without cheese) contains five hundred seventy-six calories. More than 50% of those calories come from fat. Therefore, eating habits of obese people often result in increased risk of diabetes and coronary artery disease at a young age. In essence, Ronald McDonald is not a symbol of innocence; he is a symbol of obesity, heart disease, cancer and premature death. These foods lack minerals such as chromium, vanadium, and magnesium that are required for a healthy body and for burning fat. People who are obese are actually starving themselves. This seemingly paradoxical statement reflects the inherent contradiction in trying to lose weight. Amidst a cornucopia of plenty—fruits, vegetables, lean protein sources—their body is telling them they're starving.

Another reason obese people struggle to lose weight is because they are usually depressed and anxious, and to compensate they consume more carbohydrate-rich foods to elevate their mood. And finally, because of nutrient depletions, their bodies think they are starving and send signals to the brain to eat more food. Additionally, the stress they're under from the nutrient depletions and their emotional state stimulates the secretion of cortisol in the adrenal glands. Cortisol acts to increase sugar in the blood stream, and, when there is an excess of sugar, the body turns it into fat.

This situation is what the authors call *the fat trap*. Our society unfortunately views obesity as a fault with a person's willpower. That oversimplification is not just unrealistic, it's cruel. Sugar causes a release of serotonin in the brain, which elevates mood.[184] So someone who is depressed reaches for sugar to comfort them, which is why sweets and high-carbohydrate foods are often considered comfort foods. This is a vicious cycle: as someone gets more obese and depressed, they reach for more sweets in a completely futile attempt to lift themselves out of their depression.

Another reason for obesity is lack of exercise. Obese people face several barriers when it comes to exercising. One is that they are depressed and anxious. Another is that they have difficulty physically moving. Third, they are socially ostracized so that going to a gym makes them feel self-conscious and more depressed. Also, people who want to exercise may not be able to do aerobic exercise because the excess force on their joints can be painful and can cause further degenerative joint disease.

While all of this information is important for understanding why obese people face a difficult situation, it is not a justification. The authors wish to be very blunt here—increased weight causes premature death and is a major public health hazard. Once again, it's a vicious cycle of addiction. This time it's a food addiction.

There are no easy solutions to weight problems. Popular fad diets, no matter what they're called, do not usually work. They result in a yo-yo effect on weight. People starve themselves more, lose some weight, but once they go off the diet they usually put on more weight than they lost to begin with. The major problem with diets is that they do not teach people how to eat for life. There is no magic here. People *must* consume fewer calories; the calories they do consume must be nutrient dense; and they must exercise. They also need to learn how to eat healthy to promote their overall health instead of merely focusing on short-term weight goals. Their body's biochemistry must be realigned. The best way to do this is through a combination of healthy eating and a customized program that contains nutrients for the person's unique biochemistry.

CHAPTER TWELVE

Sexual Dysfunction

A healthy sex life, one that consists of consensual sexual encounters that leave each person feeling happy and fulfilled, is an important aspect of overall health. Each partner must feel as if his or her sexual desire, called *libido*, has been satisfied.

The act of sex in and of itself does not constitute a healthy sex life. The parameters for sexual satisfaction include respect, desire, and most importantly, trust in oneself and in one's partner. The concept of trust is an extremely emotionally loaded one because it entails the notion that each person recognizes and respects the other person's verbally stated and nonverbally communicated boundaries. For a healthy sexual relationship, both partners must be physically and emotionally capable to engage in some form of sexual activity.

The psychological aspects of sexual arousal are crucial, but both people must be physically ready as well. Men must be able to have full penile tumescence (erection) for a sufficiently long enough time to be able to satisfy their partner. Similarly, women must be able to create and sustain vaginal lubrication.

One of the major problems creating an unhealthful sexual life is the fact that one or another partner, or more commonly both partners, may have decreased libido. In lay terms, the sexual desire is not there for several reasons. The most important reason for not desiring any form of sex is due to functional nutritional deficiencies in vitamins and minerals. The most common deficiency in menstruating women is iron, and lack of iron causes lassitude. Additionally, men and women are at high risk for magnesium deficiencies because of poor diets. Magnesium is a smooth muscle relaxant, and the walls of blood vessels are comprised of smooth muscle.[185-188] Magnesium therefore allows vasodilation (relaxation of blood vessel) in the pelvic region so that more blood can flow to the sexual organs for erections in men and sexual arousal in women. Nitric oxide (NO), which is produced from the essential amino acid arginine, is also required for vasodilation, and may be helpful in helping men attain betters erections.[189]

Medications for erectile dysfunction are simply vasodilators that work by increasing nitric oxide production. These medications include sildenafil (Viagra) and tadalafil (Cialis). They have been shown to temporarily improve erectile function in men but do so with risks. While these medications increase blood flow to the penis, they decrease blood flow to the eyes and may cause sudden loss of eyesight. They can also cause a drop in blood pressure (hypotension), and in men with already-decreased blood flow to the heart from coronary artery disease or congestive heart failure, they may induce a heart attack (myocardial infarction).

In the authors' opinion, working with the body's biochemical pathways to increase the body's own production of nitric oxide is in most cases an effective and safer approach than taking pharmaceutical drugs. Asymmetric dimethyl arginine (ADMA) is a protein in the body that is made from arginine.[190] Arginine can be metabolized to NO or ADMA. While NO increases blood vessel dilation, ADMA does not. Therefore, if someone is predisposed to creating ADMA instead of NO, they may develop hypertension. A blood test can detect both ADMA and arginine. If ADMA is high or arginine is low, arginine can be prescribed to push the pathway in the direction of creating NO and decreasing blood pressure, relaxing blood vessels, and increasing blood flow to the penis and vagina.

Many diseases such as cancer and diabetes can impede the circulation to either the penis or vagina. Homocysteine, which also damages blood vessels, can decrease blood flow to the sex organs. Similarly, the use of alcohol for relaxation often leads to a decreased ability to perform sexually because as Shakespeare once said in Macbeth, "The will is there but not the way." So, just as we have discussed obesity, drugs, and alcoholism, sexual performance or the lack of it becomes part of a vicious cycle of continual disappointment if one does not address the principal underlying physical and emotional issues.

Feeling relaxed and comfortable is vital for sexual arousal since the nervous system is also involved in coordinating sexual activity. If someone is nervous, it activates the sympathetic nervous system, which decreases blood flow to the penis and vagina. Alternately, relaxation stimulates the parasympathetic nervous system, which increases blood flow to the pelvis and sex organs.

Chapter Thirteen

Seizures

Seizures are excessive and abnormal electrical discharges in the brain. They can result in changes in mental state, jerking movements, and convulsions. In *petit mal* seizures, a person may appear disassociated and not recall that their seizure activity occurred at all. They do not show outward signs such as convulsions. In *grand mal* seizures, a person may collapse and have convulsions. This is the stereotypic seizure where someone is at risk of biting off their tongue and hitting their head.

The conventional diagnostic approach for seizures is to test brainwave activity using an electroencephalogram (EEG). With this device, the site of abnormal brain activity can be pinpointed. Treatment consists of anti-seizure medications such as valproic acid (Depacon, Depakene, Depakene syrup, Depakote, Depakote ER, Depakote Sprinkle, Divalproex sodium), phenytoin (Dilantin), topiramate (Topamax), gabapentin (Neurontin), and lamotrigine (Lamictal). All anti-seizure medications, however, carry serious risks for side effects, including liver damage, mitochondrial damage, gingival hyperplasia (thickening of the gums), anemia, ataxia (imbalance), lethargy, and irritability.

While the underlying causes of seizures have been studied extensively, many questions remain. Fortunately, nutritional medicine already recognizes much helpful information. One trigger for seizures is low blood sugar (hypoglycemia).[191-193] Thus, ensuring correct blood sugar control is part of a proper evaluation and treatment strategy. People can have difficulty regulating their blood sugar due to low chromium, vanadium, and essential amino acids such as threonine. An improper diet that contains high amounts of carbohydrates can also contribute to hypoglycemia. A high-carbohydrate meal or snack, such as a candy bar, soda pop, or even some yogurt with sugar added, causes a rapid increase in blood sugar levels. This stimulates a release of excessive amounts of insulin to decrease the blood sugar by facilitating its uptake by cells, but the elevated insulin can cause a drop in blood sugar that falls below a healthy level and induces hypoglycemia. This is called *reactive hypoglycemia*.[194, 195] Ensuring a diet that contains complex carbohydrates (fiber) and adequate amounts of protein with each meal or snack helps regulate blood sugar and can be very effective at keeping blood sugar levels in a healthy range. Fiber helps regulate blood sugar by slowing down the speed at which sugars are absorbed into the body, thereby decreasing the after-meal spike in blood sugar. Most food protein can be converted into glucose by the body, but since this process takes some time, the glucose gets into the bloodstream at a slower, more consistent rate. That is why people with reactive hypoglycemia should eat complex carbohydrates and protein for their energy needs instead of simple carbohydrates.

Testing biochemical parameters may have additional benefits (see table 12.1). Strategies for regulating blood sugar include testing for nutritional deficiencies, providing the nutrients required for proper blood sugar control, and counseling patients on eating regular, small meals that contain protein.

Decreased concentrations of dopamine, a neurotransmitter, can also cause seizures. Dopamine is derived from the essential amino acid phenylalanine, and its pathway requires iron, biopterin, and vitamins B3 and B6. Deficiencies in any of these cofactors can cause low dopamine. Another amino acid, taurine, which is derived from methionine and requires vitamin B6 for its production, has been shown in some clinical trials to decrease

Table 12.1. Seizure activity

Enhanced by	Decreased by
Poor blood sugar control	Histidine
Stress	GABA
Anxiety	Increasing dopamine
Strobe lights	Lowering glycine
Glycine	Taurine
Ethanolamine	Vitamin B6
Glutamate	Vitamin B3
Head trauma	Biopterin
Low dopamine	Iron

seizures in people with epilepsy. Taurine stabilizes cell membranes and can inhibit overactive nerve impulses. Testing for plasma taurine and supplementing with this amino acid if deficient may be a useful strategy.

Other amino acids that are important to evaluate are histidine, glycine, serine, ethanolamine, glutamate, and gamma-amino-butyric acid (GABA). Histidine becomes histamine in the body, and histidine administration has improved the effects of anti-seizure medications and also decreased seizure activity on its own. Elevated glycine, serine, ethanolamine, and glutamate, and low GABA, have all been implicated in seizure disorders. GABA is an inhibitory neurotransmitter (decreases nerve impulse activity), and its pathway is the same one that some anti-seizure medications target. Decreasing glycine levels have resulted in reductions in seizures in children.

In conclusion, what appears to be a very dramatic neurological abnormality is in fact created by very subtle changes in biochemistry. So anyone with seizures, whether they are taking medications or not, should receive a comprehensive biochemical evaluation. To neglect this aspect of a classical neurological workup for seizures is to avoid one of the more fundamental variables governing neurological function. Unfortunately, the vast majority of clinical neurologists and physicians are completely unaware of the influence of biochemistry on the nervous system.

Chapter Fourteen

Insomnia and Sleep Apnea

Millions of people have difficulty falling and staying asleep. This is called insomnia, and it has very serious health consequences. Sleep deprivation leads to depression, anxiety, stress, memory loss, lack of coordination, and decreased productivity. There are both metabolic and anatomical reasons for insomnia.

Sleep apnea, a condition where someone stops breathing during sleep, even for a few seconds, can wake him or her up repeatedly during the night. Many people do not realize they have sleep apnea because it does not usually completely awaken them. Instead, patients tell clinicians that others report that they snore, patients looks completely tired with bags under their eyes in the morning, and they must take a nap in the afternoon. Sleep apnea decreases oxygen intake and is a risk factor for heart and pulmonary diseases.

The key to understanding treatment options for sleep apnea is the fact that conventional treatments do not address the underlying cause and are not very effective in the long run. However, published sleep apnea cases show that a potential genetic predisposition exists that decreases one's ability to utilize vitamin B1. Clinicians can order a urine test for functional vitamin B1 deficiency with which they may infer a genetic predisposition for poor vitamin B1 utilization. The solution is to provide increasing dosages of vitamin B1 while under medical supervision and tracking changes in sleeping patterns and daily energy. Anecdotal cases have shown great improvement in patients with sleep apnea using this approach. Therefore, one may not necessarily have to resort to the drastic measures such surgery or machines that force air down someone's throat.

More commonly, anxiety, decreased production of the hormone melatonin, low blood sugar, and nocturia (getting up during the night to urinate) cause insomnia. Anxiety and low melatonin often cause difficulty falling asleep while low blood sugar and nocturia wake people up during the night. Since melatonin is produced by amino acid precursors, people who sleep better after taking melatonin may in fact simply be lacking the amino acid tryptophan or the vitamins required to transform tryptophan into melatonin.

Anxiety may be situational—due to life events—and temporary. In these cases, psychological counseling and stress reduction techniques alone or in combination may be helpful in improving sleep quality. Stress reduction may include exercise, meditation, reading, and yoga. Some people may also find it helpful to purchase a CD of soothing sounds to listen to while falling asleep. Another technique, called *sleep hygiene*, may also help. Sleep hygiene refers to creating an optimal sleep environment, such as making sure the room is dark and quiet, and not watching television in bed.

If people are waking up during the night, poor blood sugar regulation may be the cause. In many cases, simply eating five grams of protein as a snack before bed can cure the insomnia by improving blood sugar control (table 13.1). If a person lacks the nutrients required for proper blood sugar regulation such as chromium and vanadium, supplementing with these nutrients may also help.

Waking up during the night to urinate can be a sign in men of prostate enlargement. While it may be prudent to discuss this with a doctor, many people—men and women alike—simply drink too much liquid too late in the day. They must then get up one or more times to empty their bladder. Stopping all liquids in the early evening or late afternoon may solve this problem and improve sleep.

Table 13.1. Protein sources and amounts

Source	Amount
Bread, whole wheat, 1 slice	3 g
Peanut butter, 1 Tbsp	4 g
Cashews, ¼ cup	5 g
Oatmeal, 1 cup	5 g
Almonds, ¼ cup	6 g
Bagel, 1 bagel	6 g
Rice, 1 cup	6 g
Soy cheese, 1 oz	6 g
Cheese, 1 oz	7 g
Egg, 1	7 g
Millet, 1 cup	8 g
Peanuts, dry roasted, ¼ cup	9 g
Pumpkin seeds, ¼ cup	9 g
Sunflower seeds, ¼ cup	9 g

Biochemical imbalances can also produce insomnia. Decreased glycine, an inhibitory neurotransmitter, and low melatonin production can also adversely affect someone's ability to sleep. Testing and treating amino acid imbalances and nutritional deficiencies that influence blood sugar regulation can rebalance a person's biochemistry and restore proper sleep patterns.

CHAPTER FIFTEEN

Cancer

Cancer is the uncontrolled growth of cells. The normal mechanisms limiting the number of times a cell can replicate are absent in cancer cells, and they rapidly divide. Cancer cells are often shaped differently from healthy cells, they do not function properly, and they can spread to many areas of the body. The mechanism for the development of cancer involves the accumulation of damage to a cell's genes (DNA). Cancer is a group of diseases classified according to the kind of fluid or tissue in which they originate or the location in the body where they first developed. In addition, some cancers are of mixed types.

Risk factors that increase a person's chance of developing a disease are well documented for cancers and include lifestyle, genetics, diet, and environmental exposures (see table 14.1). Lifestyle and environmental factors such as smoking, high-fat diet, exposure to ultraviolet light (UV radiation from the sun), or exposure to chemicals (cancer-causing substances) in the work place over long periods of time are risk factors for some adult cancers. Most children with cancer, however, are too young to have been exposed to these lifestyle factors for any extended time, and genetics likely plays a greater role.

Table 14.1. Cancer risk factors

Category	Examples
Diet	High-saturated fat, low fiber, high in processed foods and simple carbohydrates (sugar)
Lifestyle	Smoking, lack of exercise, multiple sex partners
Genetics	BRCA1, BRCA2
Hormones	Testosterone, elevated 2-hydroxyestrogen-to-16-hydroxyestrogen ratio

Environmental exposures	Pesticides, herbicides, solvents, UV radiation from the sun

While genetic predisposition for the development of cancer is important, it plays less of a role than most people realize. Genetic factors alone explain only approximately 5% of all cancers. The *BRCA1* (breast cancer gene 1) genes have been linked to the development of breast cancer, but this genetic mutation explains only about 5% of breast cancer cases in women younger than forty years old, 2% of cases in women aged forty to forty-nine years, and 1% of cases in women aged fifty to seventy years.[100]

As with most other cancers and diseases, this shows that, in terms of breast cancer risk, genetics become less important and diet and lifestyle factors become more important the longer a person lives. In fact, it's been estimated that up to 60% of cancers in the United States are related to nutritional and lifestyle factors.

Prostate cancer is the most prevalent cancer among men and the second leading cause of cancer mortality among men in the United States. This disease disproportionately affects African American men. A man's risk for developing prostate cancer increases as his age does, according to the following general rule: 50% risk at fifty years old, 60% at sixty years old, 70% at seventy years old, and so forth. The older one gets, however, the less aggressive the cancer is likely be and the less likely it is that a man will die from the prostate cancer itself versus some other cause.

The incidence of prostate cancer is 60% higher in black men than it is in white men. Compared to Asian/Pacific Islanders, black men are three times more likely to get prostate cancer and six times more likely to die from it. A review of fourteen case-controlled studies and nine cohort studies concluded that dairy intake "is one of the most consistent dietary predictors for prostate cancer in the published literature." Data from the Physicians' Health Study, in which diet and prostate cancer incidence were documented in 20,885 male physicians for eleven years, showed that those who consumed more than 2.5 servings of dairy products per day had a 34% greater risk of getting prostate cancer compared to those who consumed 0.5 servings per day.[196]

Research suggests that the reason for the increased risk of prostate cancer in African American men is that they have a higher level of circulating testosterone. Testosterone can be converted in the prostate gland to dihydrotestosterone (DHT) by the action of the enzyme 5-alpha reductase. DHT promotes prostate cancer. The herb saw palmetto (*Seronoa repens*) inhibits the production of DHT and may prove helpful in the prevention or treatment of prostate cancer, but insufficient evidence currently precludes the use of saw palmetto. In fact, saw palmetto may decrease prostate specific antigen (PSA), a test that is used to screen for prostate cancer. By decreasing PSA, saw palmetto may make it more difficult to detect this cancer.

There is also a high correlation between sexual promiscuity and prostate cancer. The greater the number and frequency of a man's sexual partners, the higher his risk becomes. The reason for this may be sexually transmitted diseases, since infections can cause irritation in cells and DNA damage.

Liver-detoxification pathways exert major influences over the risk for and development of cancers. One such pathway metabolizes estrogen. Estrogen can be metabolized predominantly via two pathways that produce 2-hydroxyestrogen (2-OHE) and 16-hydroxyestrogen (16-OHE). 2-OHE protects against the development of breast and uterine cancers while 16-OHE increases the risk. Epidemiological studies show that a low 2-to-16 hydroxyestrogen ratio (low amounts of 2-OHE and higher amounts of 16-OHE) increases a woman's risk of breast cancer by 45%.[197] This ratio can be determined by a simple urine test, and it is a much more powerful indicator of breast cancer risk than the *BRCA1* genotype because the ratio of estrogens is a *functional* indicator of what is actually happening in the body while the genotype is not functional.

The enzymes that metabolize 16-OHE are *constitutive*, meaning that they are static and cannot be modified. Therefore, if a woman's 16-OHE level is elevated, this cannot be changed. But it's the ratio of 2-OHE to 16-OHE that's important and not the absolute concentration of each individual metabolite. The 2-OHE pathway is *inducible*; its activity can be increased so that 2-OHE production can be increased. This can be accomplished by consuming higher amounts of cruciferous vegetables, such as broccoli and cauliflower, and also by taking a dietary supplement containing adequate amounts of diindolylmethane (DIM).[198] Altering this ratio may decrease a woman's risk of developing breast and uterine cancer.

Other liver-detoxification pathways and free-radical damage to DNA have also been implicated in the risk of developing cancers. A different urine test can determine the activity of the liver-detoxification pathways. It can also detect high levels of 8-hydroxy-2-deoxyguanosine, a direct indicator of damage to DNA. Nutritional biochemistry can modulate these lab values to help decrease a person's risk for developing cancer.

Other important biochemical parameters for cancer development include low vitamin D2, which increases one's risk for colorectal and breast cancer by 50%. Testing C-reactive protein (CRP), ferritin, and fibrinogen can determine the risk factor of inflammation. Additionally, elevated levels of the amino acid glutamate and toxic-metals poisoning (e.g., lead, mercury, cadmium, arsenic) are also risk factors for cancer. A comprehensive biochemical test combined with a nutritional and lifestyle evaluation can provide the most sophisticated overall evaluation for cancer risk.

CHAPTER SIXTEEN

Case Studies in Nutritional Biochemistry

The following are examples of cases seen at Montana Integrative Medicine. These patients presented an array of medical symptoms and were evaluated using the NBI Testing and Consulting Corporation biochemical tests. They related the diagnoses they received from other doctors, such as mature-onset asthma, which is the way conventional medical doctors describe shortness of breath upon physical exertion in adults. However, that particular diagnosis, like many diagnoses, does not provide any information about the underlying causes of the symptoms. Conventional medicine provides descriptive and not functional diagnoses. Nutritional biochemical testing generates a large amount of data that allows skilled interpreters to provide functional diagnoses. A functional diagnosis is a description of the underlying biochemical causes of symptoms and diseases. For example, in the case of the gentleman with mature-onset asthma (Case 1, below), his diagnosis from a nutritional biochemistry point of view was hypertyrosinemia due to low copper and high zinc.

Case 1: Hypertyrosinemia (elevated tyrosine)

This is the case of Dr. Pieczenik, the coauthor of this book. When he was sixty-two years old, he arrived at the clinic with a previous diagnosis of mature-onset, exercise-induced asthma. This condition develops in adults and results in a decreased ability to breathe during exercise or cold weather. In his case, his lungs would constrict, and his pulmonologist determined that he had a 22% deficit in oxygen. He was literally short of breath all the time. While his pulmonologist could not determine the cause of the dysfunction, he nonetheless wanted to treat it symptomatically with steroids. Steroids have been around for more than forty years, and Dr. Pieczenik could not believe that there had been no advances in medicine during that time. Steroids carry serious risks for side effects and do nothing to cure the patient. Therefore, he decided to get a second opinion.

Dr. Pieczenik heard of Dr. Neustadt's work in nutritional biochemistry and received a complete evaluation. His results showed that he had elevated tyrosine, low copper, a low copper-to-zinc ratio, and low epinephrine (figure 15.1). Tyrosine flows down its pathway to form epinephrine and requires several vitamins and minerals to do so, including copper.

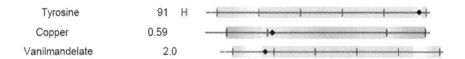

Figure 15.1. Lab results from a sixty-two-year-old male with mature onset asthma. His results show elevated tyrosine, low copper, and low vanilmandelate (VMA). VMA is a breakdown product of epinephrine, and low VMA indicates low epinephrine production.

Epinephrine is a bronchodilator (opens the airways in the lungs to increase the ability to take in oxygen), and his deficiency in epinephrine was the immediate reason why he developed mature-onset asthma. The block in the pathway was at the step where dopamine is converted to norepinephrine, which requires copper. In turn, his deficiency in copper resulted from his chronic consumption of an over-the-counter dietary supplement containing high amounts of zinc without any copper in it. He was taking fifty milligrams of zinc daily because he had read somewhere that zinc may be helpful for his prostate, but high amounts of zinc can decrease copper absorption. In effect, he induced a copper deficiency and his medical condition.

What's important here is that the evaluation identified the underlying cause of his condition, which was treatable. His conventional medical doctors would never even have known or understood the basic underlying functional biochemistry that lead to this disorder. It was never part of their medical school education and is still not taught in conventional medical programs. Instead of merely providing steroids that at best may have only relieved the symptoms, the treatment here corrected the underlying copper deficiency. Within two weeks of initiating the treatment plan to rebalance his biochemistry, the patient's mature-onset asthma was completely resolved. He did not require any steroids. In previous years, he would have left Montana in the winter for warmer climates such as Florida because the cold weather would cause bronchospasms. He now is able to stay in cold weather without any difficulties.

Case 2: Hypodopaminemia (low dopamine)

A thirty-seven-year-old male experienced seizures, life-long depression, suicidal tendencies, and extreme fatigue. This was a man who was literally at death's doorstep—he was exhausted, unable to care for himself, and without hope. His seizures began four months earlier while on a pleasure trip to Las Vegas. He had no history of head trauma or previous seizure activity. A neurologist evaluated him and ordered a computer tomography (CT) scan, a magnetic resonance imaging (MRI) study, and an electroencephalogram (EEG). All of these studies were appropriate for the medical model, and the authors of this book would have ordered them as well. However, the crucial difference between the authors' approach and a well-educated conventional neurologist is that the authors of this book would have also ordered their comprehensive nutritional biochemistry evaluation.

The conventional imaging ordered by the neurologist revealed no abnormalities. The patient was diagnosed as having "pseudo-seizures" (literally, "false seizures"), yet there was nothing false about them. The patient was prescribed different anti-seizure medications, but none reduced his seizure symptoms at all. Instead, he developed increasing depression because he felt increasingly helpless and hopeless since his symptoms were not relieved after seeing these medical experts.

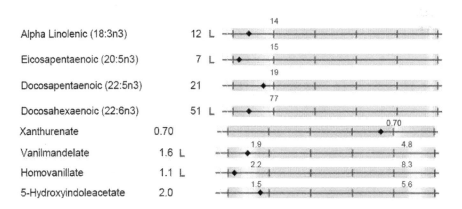

Figure 15.2. Biochemical test results for a thirty-seven-year-old male who experienced seizures, depression, and fatigue. Alpha linolenic, eicosapentaenoic, docosapentaenoic and docosahexaenoic acids are polyunsaturated fatty acids of the omega-3 series. Elevated xanthurenate is a marker for functional vitamin B6 deficiency. Low VMA, Homovanillate (HVA) and 5-Hydroxyindoleacetate are markers for low epinephrine, dopamine, and serotonin, respectively.

When he finally arrived at Montana Integrative Medicine and took the comprehensive nutritional biochemistry test, his results explained the underlying causes all of his symptoms (figure 15.2). His depression was a result of low epinephrine, low serotonin, low omega-3 fatty acids, and a functional vitamin B6 deficiency. His seizures were due to low phenylalanine, low tyrosine, low dopamine, and functionally low vitamin B6, which is required for dopamine formation. Low dopamine causes seizures and is an underlying cause of Parkinson's disease. Additionally, his medical evaluation, which included a diet recall, showed that the timing of his seizures appeared to coincide with possible low blood sugar, which is documented to cause seizures.

He was placed on a comprehensive treatment plan that included nutritional cofactors to correct his underlying biochemical dysfunction and a medically directed diet to better control his blood sugar. He was prescribed amino acids, high-dose B-vitamins, essential fatty acids, a high-quality multivitamin and mineral supplement, and a high-fiber diet. The patient's seizures stopped after being on the program for four days, and he continued to be seizure free at the three-month follow up appointment. He also reported no more depression, increased energy, no suicidal thoughts, and feeling better than he could ever remember.

Case 3: Total-Body Breakdown (TBB)

The desperate parents of a twenty-year-old female contacted the clinic to order a comprehensive nutritional biochemistry evaluation for their daughter. She had been suffering for more than eight years with progressively worse and debilitating symptoms. She experienced severe muscle weakness and spasms to the extent that she would be unable to walk for days. She was in chronic, severe pain all over her body and suffered from depression and anxiety. This young woman also experienced severe fatigue and brain fog. Every organ system in her body was dysfunctional. Although her symptoms predated the diagnosis, doctors diagnosed her with Lyme disease and administered repeated rounds of oral and intravenous antibiotics for years. They also prescribed multiple antidepressant medications and narcotics, including ever-increasing doses of methadone. All of these medical measures were merely symptomatic treatments, and she continued to deteriorate.

Her lab tests revealed deficiencies in almost every category of nutrients (amino acids, vitamins, and minerals) and biochemical pathways (figure 15.3). In short, her entire biochemistry was working improperly. This extreme and rare situation is what the authors of this book have called *total body breakdown*, which they suspect underlies the following medical diagnoses—Lyme disease, chronic fatigue syndrome, hypopituitaryism, and mitochondrial disease.

Amino-acid deficiencies			
Arginine	46 L	50 - 160	
Histidine	72	70 - 140	
Isoleucine	57	50 - 160	
Leucine	82 L	90 - 200	
Lysine	135 L	150 - 300	
Methionine	26	25 - 50	
Phenylalanine	46	45 - 140	
Threonine	152	100 - 250	
Tryptophan	34 L	35 - 65	
Valine	173	170 - 420	
Glycine	138 L	225 - 450	
Serine	94	90 - 210	
Taurine	68	50 - 250	
Tyrosine	43 L	50 - 120	
Iron-deficiency anemia			
Ferritin	4 L		
Inflammation			
c-Reactive Protein (HS)	3.7 H		
Insulin resistance			
Insulin	11.6		
Deficient essential minerals			
Chromium	0.24 L		
Copper	0.52		
Magnesium	31 L		
Manganese	0.31		
Potassium	1,415		
Selenium	0.13		
Vanadium	0.10		
Zinc	6.5		
Elevated Toxic Metal			
Arsenic	0.018		

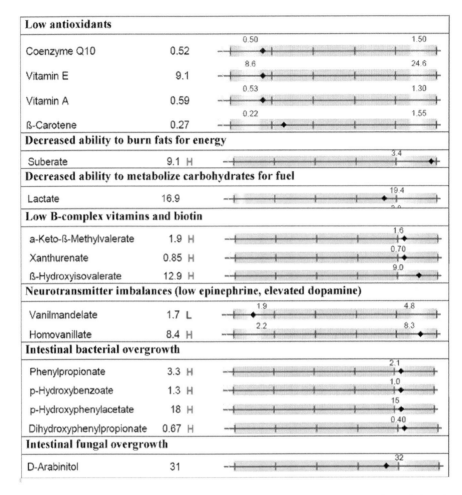

Figure 15.3. Biochemical test results for a twenty-year-old female who exhibited an eight-year history of severe depression, pain, muscle spasms, weakness, brain fog, and headaches.

This complicated case required very close management and a complex plan. Follow-up telephone consultations occurred weekly, and modifications to the plan were made as appropriate and necessary. She was placed on a comprehensive antibacterial, antifungal, and gut-rebuilding protocol for intestinal health. She began taking appropriate amino acids, vitamins, minerals, and antioxidants. Counselors also advised this woman to not push herself too hard so that her body could heal without additional stress on her systems. She began to progressively improve, and after two weeks her mother reported that at times she had her daughter back. As the weeks went on, the young woman continued to recover. She reported increased energy, improved mental acuity, decreased pain, a lifting of her depression, and a cessation of headaches. Her mother reported that it became easier to wake her daughter up in the morning and after a nap, and her daughter began getting herself out of bed in the morning and off to school without assistance. She resumed normal activities and was able to go ice-skating and to attend college.

Case 4: Age-Related Degeneration (ARD)

A sixty-nine-year-old woman suffered from extreme fatigue, weakness, muscle pain, severe gas and bloating each time she ate, and a five-year history of loose stools. When she walked less than one block, she experienced painful burning in her muscles. At the time she entered the clinic's program, she could only walk half a block and ride for one minute on a stationery bicycle. Additionally, she was unable to stand up from a seated position on the floor without assistance. She was losing strength and balance, which put her at a high risk for falling and hip fractures.

Gastroenterologists, internists, gynecologists, and urologists at major medical centers around the country had evaluated her. None of them found any abnormalities. Biochemical testing revealed deficiencies in seven out of ten amino acids, low vitamins and minerals required for mitochondrial function, an intestinal bacterial infection, and multiple food intolerances (figure 15.4).

Low amino acids		
Arginine	50	L
Histidine	65	L
Isoleucine	45	L
Leucine	85	L
Lysine	152	
Methionine	16	L
Phenylalanine	53	
Threonine	72	L
Tryptophan	43	
Valine	168	

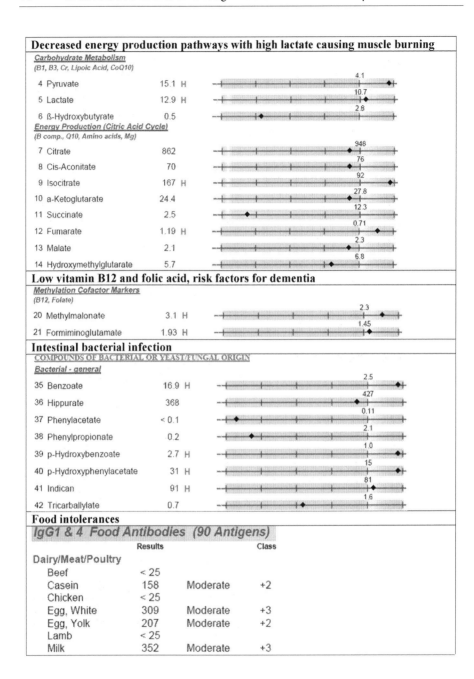

Decreased energy production pathways with high lactate causing muscle burning

Carbohydrate Metabolism
(B1, B3, Cr, Lipoic Acid, CoQ10)

4 Pyruvate	15.1 H		4.1
5 Lactate	12.9 H		10.7
6 ß-Hydroxybutyrate	0.5		2.8

Energy Production (Citric Acid Cycle)
(B comp., Q10, Amino acids, Mg)

7 Citrate	862		948
8 Cis-Aconitate	70		76
9 Isocitrate	167 H		92
10 a-Ketoglutarate	24.4		27.8
11 Succinate	2.5		12.3
12 Fumarate	1.19 H		0.71
13 Malate	2.1		2.3
14 Hydroxymethylglutarate	5.7		6.8

Low vitamin B12 and folic acid, risk factors for dementia

Methylation Cofactor Markers
(B12, Folate)

20 Methylmalonate	3.1 H		2.3
21 Formiminoglutamate	1.93 H		1.45

Intestinal bacterial infection

COMPOUNDS OF BACTERIAL OR YEAST/FUNGAL ORIGIN

Bacterial - general

35 Benzoate	16.9 H		2.5
36 Hippurate	368		427
37 Phenylacetate	< 0.1		0.11
38 Phenylpropionate	0.2		2.1
39 p-Hydroxybenzoate	2.7 H		1.0
40 p-Hydroxyphenylacetate	31 H		15
41 Indican	91 H		81
42 Tricarballylate	0.7		1.6

Food intolerances

IgG1 & 4 Food Antibodies (90 Antigens)

	Results		Class
Dairy/Meat/Poultry			
Beef	< 25		
Casein	158	Moderate	+2
Chicken	< 25		
Egg, White	309	Moderate	+3
Egg, Yolk	207	Moderate	+2
Lamb	< 25		
Milk	352	Moderate	+3

Figure 15.4. Biochemical test results for a sixty-nine-year-old woman with extreme fatigue, weakness, muscle pain, severe gas and bloating each time she ate, and a five-year history of loose stools.

Her treatment consisted of instructions to eliminate all food she showed intolerance to; to take antibacterial plant extracts for the intestinal infection; to consume a high dose of B-complex vitamins with extra vitamin B12, a customized amino acid powder, a high-quality multivitamin, and a mineral supplement; and to undergo physical therapy. Two months later, she could walk pain-free for twenty minutes twice daily and ride for ten minutes on an exercise bike. She no longer suffered from diarrhea, and her gas and bloating had also improved. Additionally, she was able to stand up from a seated position without assistance.

CHAPTER SEVENTEEN

Nosology

Nosology is a fancy term for a *system of classification*. Classification systems in medicine deal primarily with diagnosis. Unfortunately, the currently nosology used in medicine rarely describes the underlying causes. This reflects a historical bias in medicine related to descriptions of sign and symptoms. For example, the diagnosis of fatigue does not tell anything about the underlying biochemical dysfunction, and physicians are not educated in how to understand symptoms from a nutritional-biochemical perspective.

The challenge in medicine is to interview and examine patients and connect their symptoms to the underlying potential biochemical dysfunctions. Unfortunately, doctors are not educated this way, but the authors hope that this situation will change. As such, they have created a new classification system that can help the general public and physicians understand how they may use biochemical testing to create more powerful and realistic diagnoses and treatment plans.

Please do not be intimated by the tables below. The authors do not expect most readers or their doctors to necessarily understand the information. This is not a point of arrogance, but rather a point of fact that this technical information is quite complex and overwhelming to those who have not studied it. The primary reason the authors are including their nosology in the book is to establish the legitimacy of approaching medicine from a completely different perspective. Instead of viewing the body as a collection of disparate symptoms and signs with no underlying biochemical connections, as medicine does today, the authors' goal is to ultimately create a functional classification scheme that includes the complex web of biochemical interactions involved in different diseases. The authors are under no illusion that the intractable current situation in the medical system will change quickly. Like other meaningful revolutions, it will take time.

Analytes by Condition

The information in these tables is arranged alphabetically and tables are read from left-to-right across the columns.

Cardiovascular Disease Risk Factors

ADMA	Arginine
Coenzyme Q10	C-reactive protein
Direct LDL	Ferritin
Fibrinogen	Free-androgen index
HDL cholesterol	Homocysteine
Insulin	Lipid peroxides
Lipoprotein(a)	RBC magnesium
Sex-hormone-binding globulin	Testosterone
Total cholesterol	Triglycerides
Vitamin E	

Cancer Risk Factors

2/16-OH estrogen ratio	25-OH vitamin D
2-methylhippurate	8-hydroxy-2-deoxyguanosine (8-OHdG)
Aluminum	Arsenic
Cadmium	C-reactive protein
Ferritin	Fibrinogen
Lead	Low glutamine-to-glutamate ratio
Mercury	Phosphoethanolamine
p-hydroxyphenyllactate (HPLA)	Prostate-specific antigen
Putrescine	Quinolinate
Spermidine	Spermine

Depression/Fatigue

5-HIA	AA/EPA
Adipate	Alpha-keto-beta-methylvalerate
Alpha-ketoglutarate	Alpha-ketoisocaproate
Alpha-ketoisovalerate	Beta-hydroxybutyrate
Beta-hydroxyisovalerate	Celiac disease
Cis-aconitate	Citrate
Copper	Eicosapentaenoic acid
Ethanolamine	Ethylmalonate
Ferritin	Formiminoglutamate
Free T3	Fumarate
Glutamate	Glycine
Homovanillate	Hydroxymethylglutarate
IgG 1&4 food antigens	Isocitrate
Lactate	Malate
Methylmalonate	Phenylalanine
Pyruvate	Selenium
Serine	Suberate
Succinate	Taurine
Total T4	Tryptophan
Thyroid-stimulating hormone	Tyrosine
Vanilmandelate	Xanthurenate

Anxiety/Stress

5-hydroxyindoleacetate	Aluminum
Arginine	Arsenic
Cadmium	Celiac disease
Chromium	Fasting blood glucose
Ferritin	Gamma-amino butyric acid

Glycine	IgG 1&4 food antigens
Insulin	Lead
Lysine	Mercury
Threonine	Vanadium
VMA	Xanthurenate

Seizure Disorders/Parkinson's Disease

Aluminum	Arginine
Arsenic	Cadmium
Chromium	Fasting blood glucose
Histidine	Homovanillate
Isoleucine	Kynurenate
Lead	Leucine
Lysine	Mercury
Methionine	Phenylalanine
Threonine	Tryptophan
Valine	Vanadium
Xnthurenate	

Exercise-Induced and Mature-Onset Asthma

Alpha-keto-beta-methylvalarate	Alpha-ketoisocaproate
Alpha-ketoisovalerate	Copper
Ferritin	Formiminoglutamate
IgG 1&4 food antigens	Kynurenate
Methylmalonic acid	Phenylalanine
Tyrosine	Vanilmandelate
Xanthurenate	

Osteoporosis Risk and Progression

8-hydroxy-2-deoxyguanosine	Arginine
Chromium	Coenzyme Q10
Copper	C-reactive protein
Deoxypyridinoline	Ferritin
Fibrinogen	Histidine
Homocysteine	Hydroxyproline
IgG 1&4 food antigens	Isoleucine
Leucine	Lipid peroxides
Lysine	Magnesium
Methionine	Phenylalanine
Proline	Threonine
Tryptophan	Valine
Vanadium	Vitamin D
Vitamin E	Zinc

Bipolar Disorder

5-hydroxyindoleacetate	Alpha-keto-beta-methylvalarate
Alpha-ketoisocaproate	Alpha-ketoisovalerate
Beta-hydroxyisovalerate	Copper
Ethylmalonate	Fasting blood sugar
Ferritin	Formiminoglutamate
Glycine	Magnesium
Methylmalonate	Selenium
Taurine	Threonine
Xanthurenate	Zinc

Exercise Stamina

2-methylhippurate	5-hydroxyindoleacetate

Adipate	Alpha-hydroxybutyrate
Alpha-keto-beta-methylvalarate	Alpha-ketoglutarate
Alpha-ketoisocaproate	Alpha-ketoisovalerate
Aluminum	Arginine
Arsenic	Aspartic acid
Benzoate	Beta-hydroxybutyrate
Beta-hydroxyisovalerate	Cadmium
Chromium	cis-aconitate
Citrate	Citrulline
Coenzyme Q10	Copper
D-arabinitol	Dihydroxyphenylpropionate
D-lactate	Ethylmalonate
Ferritin	Formiminoglutamate
Fumarate	Glucarate
Hippurate	Histidine
Homovanillate	Hydroxymethylglutarate
IgG 1&4 food antigens	Indican
Isocitrate	Isoleucine
Kynurenate	Lactate
Lead	Leucine
Lipid peroxides	Lysine
Magnesium	Malate
Manganese	Mercury
Methionine	Methylmalonate
Orotate	Phenylacetate
Phenylalanine	Phenylpropionate
p-hydroxybenzoate	p-hydroxyphenylacetate
Potassium	Pyroglutamate
Pyruvate	Quinolinate

Selenium	Suberate
Succinate	Sulfate
Threonine	Tricarballylate
Tryptophan	Tyrosine
Valine	Vanadium
Vanilmandelate	Vitamin E
Xanthurenate	Zinc

Overweight/Obesity

2-methylhippurate	5-hydroxyindoleacetate
8-hydroxy-2'deoxyguanosine	AA/EPA
Adipate	Alpha-hydroxybutyrate
Alpha-keto-beta-methylvalarate	Alpha-ketoglutarate
Alpha-ketoisocaproate	Alpha-ketoisovalerate
Alpha-linolenic acid (ALA)	Aluminum
Arginine	Arsenic
Benzoate	Beta-hydroxybutyrate
Beta-hydroxyisovalerate	Cadmium
Chromium	cis-aconitate
Citrate	C-reactive protein
D-arabinitol	Dihydroxyphenylpropionate
D-lactate	Docosahexaenoic acid (DHA)
Dosapentaenoic acid	Eicosapentaenoic acid (EPA)
EPA/DGLA	Ethylmalonate
Ferritin	Fibrinogen
Formiminoglutamate	Free T4
Fumarate	Glucarate
Hippurate	Histidine
Homovanillate	Hydroxymethylglutarate

IgG 1&4 food antigens	Indican
Insulin	Isocitrate
Isoleucine	Kynurenate
Lactate	Lead
Leucine	Lysine
Magnesium	Malate
Manganese	Mercury
Methionine	Methylmalonate
Orotate	Percent saturation
Phenylacetate	Phenylalanine
Phenylpropionate	p-hydroxybenzoate
p-hydroxyphenylacetate	p-hydroxyphenyllactate (HPLA)
Pyroglutamate	Pyruvate
Quinolinate	Selenium
Serum iron	Suberate
Succinate	Sulfate
Threonine	Thyroid-stimulating hormone
Total-iron-binding capacity	Total T3
Tricarballylate	Triglycerides
Tryptophan	Valine
Vanadium	Vanilmandelate
Xanthurenate	Zinc

Insomnia

5-hydroxyindoleacetate	Chromium
Fasting blood glucose	Free T4
Homovanillate	Insulin
Kynurenate	Threonine
Total T3	Tryptophan

TSH	Vanadium
Vanilmandelate	Xanthurenate

Abdominal Pain

Arginine	Benzoate
D-arabinitol	Dihydroxyphenylpropionate
D-lactate	Hippurate
Histidine	Histidine
IgG 1&4 food antigens	Indican
Isoleucine	Leucine
Lysine	Methionine
Phenylacetate	Phenylalanine
Phenylpropionate	p-hydroxybenzoate
p-hydroxyphenylacetate	Threonine
Tricarballylate	Tryptophan
Valine	

Restless Leg Syndrome (RLS)

ADMA	Aluminum
Arginine	Arsenic
Cadmium	Chromium
Fasting blood glucose	Histidine
Homovanillate	Isoleucine
Kynurenate	Lead
Leucine	Lysine
Glycine	Mercury
Methionine	Phenylalanine
Threonine	Tryptophan
Valine	Tyrosine

Magnesium	Vanadium
Xanthurenate	

Muscle burning

Alpha-keto-beta-methylvalarate	Alpha-ketoisocaproate
Beta-hydroxyisovalerate	Lactate
Magnesium	Xanthurenate

Memory Loss and Dementia

8-hydroxy-2'deoxyguanosine	AA/EPA
ADMA	Alpha-keto-beta-methylvalarate
Alpha-Ketoisocaproate	Aluminum
Arginine	Arsenic
Beta-hydroxyisovalerate	Cadmium
Calcium	Chromium
Copper	C-reactive protein
EPA/DGLA	Ferritin
Fibrinogen	Glutamate
Histidine	Homocysteine
Isoleucine	Lead
Leucine	Lipid peroxides
Lysine	Magnesium
Manganese	Mercury
Methionine	Phenylalanine
Potassium	Pyroglutamate
Selenium	Threonine
Tryptophan	Valine
Vanadium	Xanthurenate
Zinc	

Autism

2-methylhippurate	5-hydroxyindoleacetate
8-hydroxy-2'deoxyguanosine	AA/EPA
Adipate	Alpha-hydroxybutyrate
Alpha-keto-beta-methylvalarate	Alpha-ketoglutarate
Alpha-ketoisocaproate	Alpha-ketoisovalerate
Aluminum	Arsenic
Asparagine	Benzoate
Beta-hydroxybutyrate	Beta-hydroxyisovalerate
Cadmium	cis-aconitate
Citrate	Cysteine
D-arabinitol	Dihydroxyphenylpropionate
D-lactate	Elevated cysteine-to-sulfate
Ethylmalonate	Formiminoglutamate
Fumarate	Gamma-amino-butyric acid
Glucarate	Glutamine
Glycine	Hippurate
Homocysteine	Homovanillate
Hydroxymethylglutarate	Indican
Isocitrate	Kynurenine
Lactate	Lead
Leucine	Lipid peroxides
Lysine	Magnesium
Malate	Mercury
Methionine	Methionine
Methylmalonate	Orotate
Phenylacetate	Phenylalanine
Phenylpropionate	p-hydroxybenzoate
p-hydroxyphenylacetate	p-hydroxyphenyllactate (HPLA)

Polyunsaturated fatty acids	Pyroglutamate
Pyroglutamate	Pyruvate
Sarcosine	Suberate
Succinate	Sulfate
Taurine	Tricarballylate
Tyrsosine	Valine
Xanthurenate	

Schizophrenia

2-methylhippurate	5-hydroxyindoleacetate
8-hydroxy-2'deoxyguanosine	Adipate
Alpha-hydroxybutyrate	Alpha-keto-beta-methylvalarate
Alpha-ketoglutarate	Alpha-ketoisocaproate
Alpha-ketoisovalerate	Aluminum
Arsenic	Benzoate
Beta-hydroxybutyrate	Beta-hydroxyisovalerate
Cadmium	Calcium
Chromium	cis-aconitate
Citrate	Copper
D-arabinitol	Dihydroxyphenylpropionate
D-lactate	Ethanolamine
Ethylmalonate	Formiminoglutamate
Fumarate	Glucarate
Glutamate	Hippurate
Homovanillate	Hydroxymethylglutarate
Indican	Isocitrate
Kynurenate	Lactate
Lead	Magnesium
Malate	Manganese

Mercury	Methylmalonate
Orotate	Phenylacetate
Phenylpropionate	p-hydroxybenzoate
p-hydroxyphenylacetate	p-hydroxyphenyllactate (HPLA)
Potassium	Pyroglutamate
Pyruvate	Quinolinate
Sarcosine	Selenium
Suberate	Succinate
Sulfate	Tricarballylate
Vanadium	Vanilmandelate
Xanthurenate	Zinc

About the Authors

John Neustadt, ND, received his naturopathic medical degree from Bastyr University. Dr. Neustadt also earned degrees in Literature (cum laude) from the University of California, San Diego, and Botany (departmental honors) from the University of Washington. He worked as a journalist in Chile and San Francisco before returning to naturopathic medical school. He is medical director of Montana Integrative Medicine and president and CEO of Nutritional Biochemistry, Incorporated (NBI) and NBI Testing and Consulting Corporation in Bozeman, Montana. Dr. Neustadt has published more than one hundred research reviews, is co-author with Jonathan Wright, MD, of the book, *Thriving through Dialysis* (Dragon Arts Publishing, Auburn, Wash, 2006), and an editor of the textbook *Laboratory Evaluations in Molecular Medicine: Nutrients, Toxicants, and Cell Regulators, 2d edition* (Metametrix, Norcross, GA, 2007).

Steve Pieczenik, MD, PhD, trained in psychiatry at Harvard and has both an MD from Cornell University Medical College and a PhD in International Relations from MIT. He is a board-certified psychiatrist and was a board examiner in psychiatry and neurology. He is chairman of the boards of NBI and NBI Testing and Consulting Corporation and an angel investor who has started more than thirty successful companies.

Contact Information

Readers may contact NBI Testing and Consulting Corporation or Montana Integrative Medicine to inquire about testing and treatment options. Additionally, the authors have created a national association, the American Association for Nutritional Biochemistry (AANB) to educate and certify other doctors in nutritional biochemistry.

NBI Testing and Consulting Corporation

1087 Stoneridge Drive, Suite 1
Bozeman, MT 59718
Toll free: 800-NBI-1416
www.nbitesting.com
info@nbitesting.com

Montana Integrative Medicine

1087 Stoneridge Drive, Suite 1
Bozeman, MT 59718
Phone: 406-582-0034
www.montanaim.com
info@montanaim.com

References

1. Gurib-Fakim A. Medicinal plants: traditions of yesterday and drugs of tomorrow. *Mol Aspects Med.* Feb 2006;27(1):1-93.

2. Ehlert U, Gaab J, Heinrichs M. Psychoneuroendocrinological contributions to the etiology of depression, posttraumatic stress disorder, and stress-related bodily disorders: the role of the hypothalamus-pituitary-adrenal axis. *Biol Psychol.* Jul-Aug 2001;57(1-3):141-152.

3. Habib KE, Gold PW, Chrousos GP. Neuroendocrinology of stress. *Endocrinol Metab Clin North Am.* Sep 2001;30(3):695-728; vii-viii.

4. Heim C, Ehlert U, Hellhammer DH. The potential role of hypocortisolism in the pathophysiology of stress-related bodily disorders. *Psych oneuroendocrinology.* Jan 2000;25(1):1-35.

5. O'Connor TM, O'Halloran DJ, Shanahan F. The stress response and the hypothalamic-pituitary-adrenal axis: from molecule to melancholia. *Qjm.* Jun 2000;93(6):323-333.

6. Shames R. Nutritional Management of Stress-Induced Dysfunction. *ANSR.* 2002(January 2002):1-7.

7. Miller ER, 3rd, Pastor-Barriuso R, Dalal D, Riemersma RA, Appel LJ, Guallar E. Meta-Analysis: High-Dosage Vitamin E Supplementation May Increase All-Cause Mortality. *Ann Intern Med.* Nov 10 2004.

8. Bjelakovic G, Nikolova D, Gluud LL, Simonetti RG, Gluud C. Mortality in Randomized Trials of Antioxidant Supplements for Primary and Secondary Prevention: Systematic Review and Meta-analysis. *JAMA.* 2007;297(8):842-857.

9. Eysenck HJ. Meta-analysis and its problems. *BMJ.* Sep 24 1994;309(6957):789-792.

10. Banks RE, Dunn MJ, Hochstrasser DF, et al. Proteomics: new perspectives, new biomedical opportunities. *Lancet.* Nov 18 2000;356(9243):1749-1756.

11. Bralley J, Lord R. Chapter 4: Amino Acids. *Laboratory Evaluations in Molecular Medicine: Nutrients, Toxicants, and Cell Regulators.* Norcross, GA: The Institute for Advances in Molecular Medicine; 2001:75-131.

12. Kure S, Hou D-C, Ohura T, et al. Tetrahydrobiopterin-responsive phenylalanine hydroxylase deficiency. *The Journal of Pediatrics.* 1999;135(3):375-378.

13. Muntau AC, Roschinger W, Habich M, et al. Tetrahydrobiopterin as an Alternative Treatment for Mild Phenylketonuria. *N Engl J Med.* 2002;347(26):2122-2132.

14. Williams R. *Biochemical Individuality: the basis for the genotrophic concept.* New York: McGraw-Hill; 1998.

15. Groff JL, Gropper SS. *Advanced Nutrition and Human Metabolism.* Third ed. Belmont: Wadsworth; 2000.

16. Ross SA, McCaffery PJ, Drager UC, De Luca LM. Retinoids in Embryonal Development. *Physiol. Rev.* 2000;80(3):1021-1054.

17. Jacob RA, Sotoudeh G. Vitamin C Function and Status in Chronic Disease. *Nutrition in Clinical Care.* 2002;5(2):66-74.

18. Hickey S, Roberts H. Misleading information on the properties of vitamin C. *PLoS Med.* Sep 2005;2(9):e307; author reply e309.

19. Cathcart RF. Vitamin C, titrating to bowel tolerance, anascorbemia, and acute induced scurvy. *Med Hypotheses.* Nov 1981;7(11):1359-1376.

20. Cathcart RF. The method of determining proper doses of vitamin C for the treatment of diseases by titrating to bowel intolerance. *Australas Nurses J.* Mar 1980;9(4):9-13.

21. Shils ME. Magnesium. In: Shils M, Olson J, A., Shike M, Ross AC, eds. *Nutrition in Health and Disease.* 9th ed. Baltimore: Williams & Wilkins; 1999:169-192.

22. Ames BN. Low micronutrient intake may accelerate the degenerative diseases of aging through allocation of scarce micronutrients by triage. *PNAS.* 2006;103(47):17589-17594.

23. Berry MJ, Larsen PR. The role of selenium in thyroid hormone action. *Endocr Rev.* May 1992;13(2):207-219.

24. Kohrle J. The deiodinase family: selenoenzymes regulating thyroid hormone availability and action. *Cell Mol Life Sci.* Dec 2000;57(13-14):1853-1863.

25. Kralik A, Eder K, Kirchgessner M. Influence of zinc and selenium deficiency on parameters relating to thyroid hormone metabolism. *Horm Metab Res.* May 1996;28(5):223-226.

26. Gaby AR. Sub-laboratory hypothyroidism and the empirical use of Armour thyroid. *Altern Med Rev.* Jun 2004;9(2):157-179.

27.   Jovanovic SV, Simic MG. Antioxidants in nutrition. *Ann N Y Acad Sci.* 2000;899:326-334.

28.   Steinberg D. Low density lipoprotein oxidation and its pathobiological significance. *J Biol Chem.* 1997;272(34):20963-20966.

29.   Aviram M, Fuhrman B. LDL oxidation by arterial wall macrophages depends on the oxidative status in the lipoprotein and in the cells: role of prooxidants vs. antioxidants. *Mol Cell Biochem.* Nov 1998;188(1-2):149-159.

30.   Mackness MI, Durrington PN, Mackness B. How high-density lipoprotein protects against the effects of lipid peroxidation. *Curr Opin Lipidol.* Aug 2000;11(4):383-388.

31.   Cestaro B, Giuliani A, Fabris F, Scarafiotti C. Free radicals, atherosclerosis, ageing and related dysmetabolic pathologies: biochemical and molecular aspects. *Eur J Cancer Prev.* Mar 1997;6 Suppl 1:S25-30.

32.   Bruckdorfer KR. Antioxidants, lipoprotein oxidation, and arterial function. *Lipids.* Mar 1996;31 Suppl:S83-85.

33.   Neustadt J. Mitochondrial dysfunction and disease. *Integr Med.* 2006;5(3):14-20.

34.   Segal AW. How Neutrophils Kill Microbes. *Annual Review of Immunology.* 2005;23(1):197-223.

35.   Ross JA, Kasum CM. Dietary flavonoids: bioavailability, metabolic effects, and safety. *Annu Rev Nutr.* 2002;22:19-34.

36.   Knekt P, Kumpulainen J, Jarvinen R, et al. Flavonoid intake and risk of chronic diseases. *Am J Clin Nutr.* Sep 2002;76(3):560-568.

37.   Bravo L. Polyphenols: chemistry, dietary sources, metabolism, and nutritional significance. *Nutr Rev.* Nov 1998;56(11):317-333.

38.   Maron DJ. Flavonoids for reduction of atherosclerotic risk. *Curr Atheroscler Rep.* Jan 2004;6(1):73-78.

39.   Donovan JL. Flavonoids and the risk of cardiovascular disease in women. *Am J Clin Nutr.* March 1, 2004 2004;79(3):522-523.

40.   Aviram M, Dornfeld L, Kaplan M, et al. Pomegranate juice flavonoids inhibit low-density lipoprotein oxidation and cardiovascular diseases: studies in atherosclerotic mice and in humans. *Drugs Exp Clin Res.* 2002;28(2-3):49-62.

41.   Vita JA. Polyphenols and cardiovascular disease: effects on endothelial and platelet function. *Am J Clin Nutr.* January 1, 2005 2005;81(1):292S-297.

42.   Arts IC, Hollman PC. Polyphenols and disease risk in epidemiologic studies. *Am J Clin Nutr.* 2005;81(1):317S-325.

43. Neustadt J. Antioxidants: Redefining Their Roles. *Integr Med.* 2006;5(6):22-26.

44. Simopoulos AP. The Mediterranean Diets: What Is So Special about the Diet of Greece? The Scientific Evidence. *J. Nutr.* 2001;131(11):3065S-3073.

45. Simopoulos AP. The importance of the ratio of omega-6/omega-3 essential fatty acids. *Biomed Pharmacother.* Oct 2002;56(8):365-379.

46. Neustadt J. The food pyramid and disease prevention. *Integr Med.* 2005;4(6):14-19.

47. Neustadt J. Western Diet and Inflammation. *Integr Med.* 2006;5(4):14-18.

48. Fung TT, Willett WC, Stampfer MJ, Manson JE, Hu FB. Dietary Patterns and the Risk of Coronary Heart Disease in Women. *Arch Intern Med.* 2001;161(15):1857-1862.

49. Cordain L, Eaton SB, Sebastian A, et al. Origins and evolution of the Western diet: health implications for the 21st century. *Am J Clin Nutr.* 2005;81(2):341-354.

50. Hasler CM. The Changing Face of Functional Foods. *J Am Coll Nutr.* 2000;19(90005):499S-506.

51. Fernandez ML. Dietary cholesterol provided by eggs and plasma lipoproteins in healthy populations. *Curr Opin Clin Nutr Metab Care.* Jan 2006;9(1):8-12.

52. Valenzuela A, Sanhueza J, Nieto S. Cholesterol oxidation: health hazard and the role of antioxidants in prevention. *Biol Res.* 2003;36(3-4):291-302.

53. Hubbard RW, Ono Y, Sanchez A. Atherogenic effect of oxidized products of cholesterol. *Prog Food Nutr Sci.* 1989;13(1):17-44.

54. Mutanen M, Freese R. Fats, lipids and blood coagulation. *Curr Opin Lipidol.* Feb 2001;12(1):25-29.

55. Harbige LS. Dietary n-6 and n-3 fatty acids in immunity and autoimmune disease. *Proc Nutr Soc.* Nov 1998;57(4):555-562.

56. Lichtenstein AH. Dietary fat and cardiovascular disease risk: quantity or quality? *J Womens Health (Larchmt).* Mar 2003;12(2):109-114.

57. Campbell TC. *The China Study.* Dallas, TX: Benbella Books; 2005.

58. Worthington V. Nutritional quality of organic versus conventional fruits, vegetables and grains. *Journal of Alternative and Complementary Medicine.* 2001;7(2):161-173.

59. Reddy MB, Love M. The impact of food processing on the nutritional quality of vitamins and minerals. *Adv Exp Med Biol.* 1999;459:99-106.

60. Agte V, Tarwadi K, Mengale S, Hinge A, Chiplonkar S. Vitamin profile of cooked foods: how healthy is the practice of ready-to-eat foods? *Int J Food Sci Nutr.* May 2002;53(3):197-208.

61. Nesheim RO. Nutrient changes in food processing. A current review. *Fed Proc.* Nov 1974;33(11):2267-2269.

62. Schroeder HA. Losses of vitamins and trace minerals resulting from processing and preservation of foods. *Am J Clin Nutr.* May 1971;24(5):562-573.

63. Bralley J, Lord R. *Laboratory Evaluations in Molecular Medicine: Nutrients, Toxicants, and Cell Regulators.* Norcross, GA: The Institute for Advances in Molecular Medicine; 2001.

64. Kirjavainen PV, Gibson GR. Healthy gut microflora and allergy: factors influencing development of the microbiota. *Ann Med.* Aug 1999;31(4):288-292.

65. Barbeau WE. Interactions between dietary proteins and the human system: implications for oral tolerance and food-related diseases. *Adv Exp Med Biol.* 1997;415:183-193.

66. Stanley S. Oral tolerance of food. *Curr Allergy Asthma Rep.* Jan 2002;2(1):73-77.

67. Schneeman BO. Gastrointestinal physiology and functions. *Br J Nutr.* Nov 2002;88 Suppl 2:S159-163.

68. Hurwitz A, Brady DA, Schaal SE, Samloff IM, Dedon J, Ruhl CE. Gastric acidity in older adults. *Jama.* Aug 27 1997;278(8):659-662.

69. Kassarjian Z, Russell RM. Hypochlorhydria: A Factor in Nutrition. *Annual Review of Nutrition.* 1989;9(1):271-285.

70. Wood RJ, Suter PM, Russell RM. Mineral requirements of elderly people. *Am J Clin Nutr.* 1995;62(3):493-505.

71. Baik HW, Russell RM. Vitamin B12 deficiency in the elderly. *Annu Rev Nutr.* 1999;19:357-377.

72. Prousky JE. Cobalamin deficiency in elderly patients. *CMAJ.* 2005;172(4):450-a-451.

73. Sturniolo GC, Montino MC, Rossetto L, et al. Inhibition of gastric acid secretion reduces zinc absorption in man. *J Am Coll Nutr.* Aug 1991;10(4):372-375.

74. Kelly GS. Hydrochloric Acid: Physiological Functions and Clinical Implications. *Alt Med Rev.* 1997;2(2):116-127.

75. Sharp GS. The diagnosis and treatment of achlorhydria; preliminary report of new simplified methods. *West J Surg Obstet Gynecol.* Jul 1953;61(7):353-360.

76.   Yang YX, Lewis JD, Epstein S, Metz DC. Long-term proton pump inhibitor therapy and risk of hip fracture. *JAMA.* 2006;296(24):2947-2953.

77.   Martinsen TC, Bergh K, Waldum HL. Gastric juice: a barrier against infectious diseases. *Basic Clin Pharmacol Toxicol.* Feb 2005;96(2):94-102.

78.   Hongo M, Ishimori A, Nagasaki A, Sato T. Effect of duodenal acidification on the lower esophageal sphincter pressure in the dog with special reference to related gastrointestinal hormones. *Tohoku J Exp Med.* Jul 1980;131(3):215-219.

79.   Wright JV. *Dr. Wright's Guide to Healing with Nutrition.* New Canaan, CT: Keats Publishing; 1990.

80.   Simon GL, Gorbach SL. Intestinal flora in health and disease. *Gastroenterology.* Jan 1984;86(1):174-193.

81.   Guarner F, Malagelada J-R. Gut flora in health and disease. *The Lancet.* 2003;361(9356):512-519.

82.   Bengmark S. Ecological control of the gastrointestinal tract. The role of probiotic flora. *Gut.* Jan 1998;42(1):2-7.

83.   Urita Y, Sugimoto M, Hike K, et al. High incidence of fermentation in the digestive tract in patients with reflux oesophagitis. *Eur J Gastroenterol Hepatol.* May 2006;18(5):531-535.

84.   Tomohiko S, Masaki I, Nobue H, Yoko H, Masuo N, Susumu T. Gastric Acid Normosecretion Is Not Essential in the Pathogenesis of Mild Erosive Gastroesophageal Reflux Disease in Relation to Helicobacter pylori Status. *Digestive Diseases and Sciences.* 2004;V49(5):787-794.

85.   Gershon M. *The Second Brain: A Groundbreaking New Understanding of Nervous Disorders of the Stomach and Intestine.* New York: Harper; 1999.

86.   Santos J, Bayarri C, Saperas E, et al. Characterisation of immune mediator release during the immediate response to segmental mucosal challenge in the jejunum of patients with food allergy. *Gut.* 1999;45(4):553-558.

87.   Rodrigo L. Celiac disease. *World J Gastroenterol.* Nov 7 2006;12(41):6585-6593.

88.   Hernandez L, Green PH. Extraintestinal manifestations of celiac disease. *Curr Gastroenterol Rep.* Oct 2006;8(5):383-389.

89.   Hvatum M, Kanerud L, Hallgren R, Brandtzaeg P. The gut-joint axis: cross reactive food antibodies in rheumatoid arthritis. *Gut.* 2006;55(9):1240-1247.

90.   Zar S, Kumar D, Benson MJ. Food hypersensitivity and irritable bowel syndrome. *Alimentary Pharmacology & Therapeutics.* 2001;15(4):439-449.

91.   Rowntree S, Platts-Mills TA, Cogswell JJ, Mitchell EB. A subclass IgG4-specific antigen-binding radioimmunoassay (RIA): comparison between IgG and IgG4 antibodies to food and inhaled antigens in adult atopic dermatitis after desensitization treatment and during development of antibody responses in children. *J Allergy Clin Immunol.* Oct 1987;80(4):622-630.

92.   Calkhoven PG, Aalbers M, Koshte VL, et al. Relationship between IgG1 and IgG4 antibodies to foods and the development of IgE antibodies to inhalant allergens. II. Increased levels of IgG antibodies to foods in children who subsequently develop IgE antibodies to inhalant allergens. *Clin Exp Allergy.* Jan 1991;21(1):99-107.

93.   Christenson JG, Dairman W, Udenfriend S. On the identity of DOPA decarboxylase and 5-hydroxytryptophan decarboxylase (immunological titration-aromatic L-amino acid decarboxylase-serotonin-dopamine-norepinephrine). *Proc Natl Acad Sci U S A.* Feb 1972;69(2):343-347.

94.   Garrod AE. The incidence of alkaptonuria: a study in chemical individuality. *The Lancet.* 1902;11:1616-1620.

95.   Ames BN. The metabolic tune-up: metabolic harmony and disease prevention. *J Nutr.* May 2003;133(5 Suppl 1):1544S-1548S.

96.   Ames BN. Delaying the Mitochondrial Decay of Aging. *Ann NY Acad Sci.* 2004;1019(1):406-411.

97.   Ames BN, Atamna H, Killilea DW. Mineral and vitamin deficiencies can accelerate the mitochondrial decay of aging. *Mol Aspects Med.* 2005;26(4-5):363-378.

98.   Ames BN, Elson-Schwab I, Silver EA. High-dose vitamin therapy stimulates variant enzymes with decreased coenzyme binding affinity (increased K(m)): relevance to genetic disease and polymorphisms. *Am J Clin Nutr.* Apr 2002;75(4):616-658.

99.   Ames BN, Shigenaga MK, Hagen TM. Oxidants, antioxidants, and the degenerative diseases of aging. *Proc Natl Acad Sci U S A.* Sep 1 1993;90(17):7915-7922.

100.   Rock CL, Lampe JW, Patterson RE. Nutrition, Genetics, and Risks of Cancer. *Annual Review of Public Health.* 2000;21(1):47-64.

101.   Seashore MR. Tetrahydrobiopterin and Dietary Restriction in Mild Phenylketonuria. *N Engl J Med.* 2002;347(26):2094-2095.

102.   van Meurs JBJ, Dhonukshe-Rutten RAM, Pluijm SMF, et al. Homocysteine Levels and the Risk of Osteoporotic Fracture. *N Engl J Med.* 2004;350(20):2033-2041.

103.   Rimm EB, Willett WC, Hu FB, et al. Folate and Vitamin B6 From Diet and Supplements in Relation to Risk of Coronary Heart Disease Among Women. *JAMA.* 1998;279(5):359-364.

104.   Kim Y-I. Nutritional Epigenetics: Impact of Folate Deficiency on DNA Methylation and Colon Cancer Susceptibility. *J. Nutr.* 2005;135(11):2703-2709.

105.   Klerk M, Verhoef P, Clarke R, Blom HJ, Kok FJ, Schouten EG. MTHFR 677C—>T polymorphism and risk of coronary heart disease: a meta-analysis. *Jama.* Oct 23-30 2002;288(16):2023-2031.

106.   Brown AA, Hu FB. Dietary modulation of endothelial function: implications for cardiovascular disease. *Am J Clin Nutr.* 2001;73(4):673-686.

107.   Ravaglia G, Forti P, Maioli F, et al. Homocysteine and cognitive function in healthy elderly community dwellers in Italy. *Am J Clin Nutr.* 2003;77(3):668-673.

108.   Seshadri S, Beiser A, Selhub J, et al. Plasma homocysteine as a risk factor for dementia and Alzheimer's disease. *N Engl J Med.* Feb 14 2002;346(7):476-483.

109.   Welch GN, Loscalzo J. Homocysteine and Atherothrombosis. *N Engl J Med.* 1998;338(15):1042-1050.

110.   Spees JL, Olson SD, Whitney MJ, Prockop DJ. Mitochondrial transfer between cells can rescue aerobic respiration. *PNAS.* 2006;103(5):1283-1288.

111.   DiMauro S, Schon EA. Mitochondrial Respiratory-Chain Diseases. *N Engl J Med.* June 26, 2003 2003;348(26):2656-2668.

112.   Luft R, Ikkos D, Palmieri G, Ernster L, Afzelius B. A case of severe hypermetabolism of nonthyroid origin with a defect in the maintenance of mitochondrial respiratory control: a correlated clinical, biochemical, and morphological study. *J Clin Invest.* Sep 1962;41:1776-1804.

113.   Wallace DC. A mitochondrial paradigm of metabolic and degenerative diseases, aging, and cancer: A dawn for evolutionary medicine. *Annual Review of Genetics.* 2005;39(1):359-407.

114.   Fosslien E. Mitochondrial Medicine—Molecular Pathology of Defective Oxidative Phosphorylation. *Ann Clin Lab Sci.* 2001;31(1):25-67.

115. West IC. Radicals and oxidative stress in diabetes. *Diabet Med.* Mar 2000;17(3):171-180.

116. Stavrovskaya IG, Kristal BS. The powerhouse takes control of the cell: Is the mitochondrial permeability transition a viable therapeutic target against neuronal dysfunction and death? *Free Radical Biology and Medicine.* 2005;38(6):687-697.

117. Koike K. Molecular basis of hepatitis C virus-associated hepatocarcinogenesis: lessons from animal model studies. *Clin Gastroenterol Hepatol.* Oct 2005;3(10 Suppl 2):S132-135.

118. Stork C, Renshaw PF. Mitochondrial dysfunction in bipolar disorder: evidence from magnetic resonance spectroscopy research. *Mol Psychiatry.* Oct 2005;10(10):900-919.

119. Fattal O, Budur K, Vaughan AJ, Franco K. Review of the literature on major mental disorders in adult patients with mitochondrial diseases. *Psychosomatics.* Jan-Feb 2006;47(1):1-7.

120. Savitha S, Sivarajan K, Haripriya D, Kokilavani V, Panneerselvam C. Efficacy of levo carnitine and alpha lipoic acid in ameliorating the decline in mitochondrial enzymes during aging. *Clin Nutr.* 2005;24(5):794-800.

121. Skulachev VP, Longo VD. Aging as a mitochondria-mediated atavistic program: can aging be switched off? *Ann N Y Acad Sci.* Dec 2005;1057:145-164.

122. Corral-Debrinski M, Shoffner JM, Lott MT, Wallace DC. Association of mitochondrial DNA damage with aging and coronary atherosclerotic heart disease. *Mutat Res.* Sep 1992;275(3-6):169-180.

123. Einat H, Yuan P, Manji HK. Increased anxiety-like behaviors and mitochondrial dysfunction in mice with targeted mutation of the Bcl-2 gene: further support for the involvement of mitochondrial function in anxiety disorders. *Behav Brain Res.* Dec 7 2005;165(2):172-180.

124. Lieber CS, Leo MA, Mak KM, et al. Model of nonalcoholic steatohepatitis. *Am J Clin Nutr.* 2004;79(3):502-509.

125. Puddu P, Puddu GM, Galletti L, Cravero E, Muscari A. Mitochondrial dysfunction as an initiating event in atherogenesis: a plausible hypothesis. *Cardiology.* 2005;103(3):137-141.

126. Bua EA, McKiernan SH, Wanagat J, McKenzie D, Aiken JM. Mitochondrial abnormalities are more frequent in muscles undergoing sarcopenia. *J Appl Physiol.* 2002;92(6):2617-2624.

127.   Conley KE, Esselman PC, Jubrias SA, et al. Ageing, muscle properties and maximal O(2) uptake rate in humans. *J Physiol.* Jul 1 2000;526 Pt 1:211-217.

128.   Buist R. Elevated Xenobiotics, Lactate and Pyruvate in C.F.S. Patients. *Journal of Orthomolecular Medicine.* 1989;4(3):170-172.

129.   Park JH, Niermann KJ, Olsen N. Evidence for metabolic abnormalities in the muscles of patients with fibromyalgia. *Curr Rheumatol Rep.* Apr 2000;2(2):131-140.

130.   Yunus MB, Kalyan-Raman UP, Kalyan-Raman K. Primary fibromyalgia syndrome and myofascial pain syndrome: clinical features and muscle pathology. *Arch Phys Med Rehabil.* Jun 1988;69(6):451-454.

131.   Veltri KL, Espiritu M, Singh G. Distinct genomic copy number in mitochondria of different mammalian organs. *J Cell Physiol.* Apr 1990;143(1):160-164.

132.   Gray MW. Origin and evolution of mitochondrial DNA. *Annu Rev Cell Biol.* 1989;5:25-50.

133.   Aw TY, Jones DP. Nutrient Supply and Mitochondrial Function. *Annual Review of Nutrition.* 1989;9(1):229-251.

134.   Chance B, Sies H, Boveris A. Hydroperoxide metabolism in mammalian organs. *Physiol Rev.* Jul 1979;59(3):527-605.

135.   Chan K, Truong D, Shangari N, O'Brien PJ. Drug-induced mitochondrial toxicity. *Expert Opin Drug Metab Toxicol.* Dec 2005;1(4):655-669.

136.   Fromenty B, Pessayre D. Impaired mitochondrial function in microvesicular steatosis effects of drugs, ethanol, hormones and cytokines. *Journal of Hepatology.* 1997;26(Supplement 2):43-53.

137.   Chitturi SMD, George JPD. Hepatotoxicity of Commonly Used Drugs: Nonsteroidal Anti-Inflammatory Drugs, Antihypertensives, Antidiabetic Agents, Anticonvulsants, Lipid-Lowering Agents, Psychotropic Drugs. *Seminars in Liver Disease.* 2002(2):169-184.

138.   Modica-Napolitano JS, Lagace CJ, Brennan WA, Aprille JR. Differential effects of typical and atypical neuroleptics on mitochondrial function in vitro. *Arch Pharm Res.* Nov 2003;26(11):951-959.

139.   Balijepalli S, Kenchappa RS, Boyd MR, Ravindranath V. Protein thiol oxidation by haloperidol results in inhibition of mitochondrial complex I in brain regions: comparison with atypical antipsychotics. *Neurochem Int.* Apr 2001;38(5):425-435.

140. Balijepalli S, Boyd MR, Ravindranath V. Inhibition of mitochondrial complex I by haloperidol: the role of thiol oxidation. *Neuropharmacology.* Apr 1999;38(4):567-577.

141. Maurer I, Moller HJ. Inhibition of complex I by neuroleptics in normal human brain cortex parallels the extrapyramidal toxicity of neuroleptics. *Mol Cell Biochem.* Sep 1997;174(1-2):255-259.

142. Kalivas PW, Volkow ND. The Neural Basis of Addiction: A Pathology of Motivation and Choice. *Am J Psychiatry.* 2005;162(8):1403-1413.

143. Volkow ND, Fowler JS, Wang GJ, Swanson JM. Dopamine in drug abuse and addiction: results from imaging studies and treatment implications. *Mol Psychiatry.* Jun 2004;9(6):557-569.

144. Wang GJ, Volkow ND, Thanos PK, Fowler JS. Similarity between obesity and drug addiction as assessed by neurofunctional imaging: a concept review. *J Addict Dis.* 2004;23(3):39-53.

145. Lydeking-Olsen E, Beck-Jensen JE, Setchell KD, Holm-Jensen T. Soymilk or progesterone for prevention of bone loss: a 2 year randomized, placebo-controlled trial. *Eur J Nutr.* Aug 2004;43(4):246-257.

146. Weisman SM, Matkovic V. Potential use of biochemical markers of bone turnover for assessing the effect of calcium supplementation and predicting fracture risk. *Clinical Therapeutics.* 2005;27(3):299-308.

147. Gaby AR. Diagnostic tests for osteoporosis. *Townsend Letters for Doctors and Patients.* October 31 1998.

148. Hara K, Kobayashi M, Akiyama Y. Vitamin K2 (menatetrenone) inhibits bone loss induced by prednisolone partly through enhancement of bone formation in rats. *Bone.* Nov 2002;31(5):575-581.

149. Sato Y, Kanoko T, Satoh K, Iwamoto J. Menatetrenone and vitamin D2 with calcium supplements prevent nonvertebral fracture in elderly women with Alzheimer's disease. *Bone.* 2005;36(1):61-68.

150. Sato Y, Honda Y, Kaji M, et al. Amelioration of osteoporosis by menatetrenone in elderly female Parkinson's disease patients with vitamin D deficiency. *Bone.* 2002/7 2002;31(1):114-118.

151. Purwosunu Y, Rachman IA, Reksoprodjo S, Sekizawa A. Vitamin K2 treatment for postmenopausal osteoporosis in Indonesia. *Journal of Obstetrics and Gynaecology Research.* 2006;32(2):230-234.

152. Shiraki M, Shiraki Y, Aoki C, Miura M. Vitamin K2 (Menatetrenone) Effectively Prevents Fractures and Sustains Lumbar Bone Mineral Density in Osteoporosis. *Journal of Bone and Mineral Research.* 2000;15(3):515-522.

153.   Iwamoto J, Takeda T, Ichimura S. Effect of combined administration of vitamin D3 and vitamin K2 on bone mineral density of the lumbar spine in postmenopausal women with osteoporosis. *J Orthop Sci.* 2000;5(6):546-551.

154.   Iwamoto I, Kosha S, Noguchi S-i, et al. A longitudinal study of the effect of vitamin K2 on bone mineral density in postmenopausal women a comparative study with vitamin D3 and estrogen-progestin therapy. *Maturitas.* 1999;31(2):161-164.

155.   Ushiroyama T, Ikeda A, Ueki M. Effect of continuous combined therapy with vitamin K2 and vitamin D3 on bone mineral density and coagulofibrinolysis function in postmenopausal women. *Maturitas.* 2002;41(3):211-221.

156.   Bischoff-Ferrari HA, Willett WC, Wong JB, Giovannucci E, Dietrich T, Dawson-Hughes B. Fracture Prevention With Vitamin D Supplementation: A Meta-analysis of Randomized Controlled Trials. *JAMA.* 2005;293(18):2257-2264.

157.   Trivedi DP, Doll R, Khaw KT. Effect of four monthly oral vitamin D3 (cholecalciferol) supplementation on fractures and mortality in men and women living in the community: Randomised double blind controlled trial. *British Medical Journal.* 2003;326(7387):469-472.

158.   Rose WC, Haines WJ, Warner DT. The amino acid requirements of man. V. The role of lysine, arginine, and tryptophan. *J Biol Chem.* Jan 1954;206(1):421-430.

159.   Rose WC, Warner DT, Haines WJ. The amino acid requirements of man. IV. The role of leucine and phenylalanine. *J Biol Chem.* Dec 1951;193(2):613-620.

160.   Rose WC, Haines WJ, Warner DT. The amino acid requirements of man. III. The role of isoleucine; additional evidence concerning histidine. *J Biol Chem.* Dec 1951;193(2):605-612.

161.   Rose WC, Haines WJ, Warner DT, Johnson JE. The amino acid requirements of man. II. The role of threonine and histidine. *J Biol Chem.* Jan 1951;188(1):49-58.

162.   Mohseni S. Hypoglycemic neuropathy. *Acta Neuropathol (Berl).* Nov 2001;102(5):413-421.

163.   DeBellis R, Smith BS, Choi S, Malloy M. Management of delirium tremens. *J Intensive Care Med.* May-Jun 2005;20(3):164-173.

164.   Bayard M, McIntyre J, Hill KR, Woodside J, Jr. Alcohol withdrawal syndrome. *Am Fam Physician.* Mar 15 2004;69(6):1443-1450.

165. Katan MB, Schouten E. Caffeine and arrhythmia. *Am J Clin Nutr.* 2005;81(3):539-540.

166. Cook JD, Lipschitz DA, Miles LE, Finch CA. Serum ferritin as a measure of iron stores in normal subjects. *Am J Clin Nutr.* Jul 1974;27(7):681-687.

167. Cook JD, Skikne BS. Iron deficiency: definition and diagnosis. *J Intern Med.* Nov 1989;226(5):349-355.

168. Kostaropoulos IA, Nikolaidis MG, Jamurtas AZ, et al. Comparison of the blood redox status between long-distance and short-distance runners. *Physiol Res.* 2006;55(6):611-616.

169. Dementia. *The Merck Manual of Geriatrics* [http://www.merck.com/mrkshared/mmg/sec5/ch40/ch40a.jsp. Accessed March 9, 2007].

170. Casademont J, Miro O, Rodriguez-Santiago B, Viedma P, Blesa R, Cardellach F. Cholinesterase inhibitor rivastigmine enhance the mitochondrial electron transport chain in lymphocytes of patients with Alzheimer's disease. *J Neurol Sci.* Jan 15 2003;206(1):23-26.

171. Liang Y-q, Tang X-c. Comparative studies of huperzine A, donepezil, and rivastigmine on brain acetylcholine, dopamine, norepinephrine, and 5-hydroxytryptamine levels in freely-moving rats. *Acta Pharmacologica Sinica.* 2006;27(9):1127-1136.

172. Wang R, Yan H, Tang X-c. Progress in studies of huperzine A, a natural cholinesterase inhibitor from Chinese herbal medicine. *Acta Pharmacologica Sinica.* 1;27(1):1-26.

173. Higdon J. Choline. *Micronutrient Information Center* [http://lpi.oregonstate.edu/infocenter/othernuts/choline/. Accessed March 9, 2007].

174. de Quervain DJF, Henke K, Aerni A, et al. Glucocorticoid-induced impairment of declarative memory retrieval is associated with reduced blood flow in the medial temporal lobe. *European Journal of Neuroscience.* 2003;17(6):1296-1302.

175. de Leon MJ, McRae T, Rusinek H, et al. Cortisol Reduces Hippocampal Glucose Metabolism in Normal Elderly, but Not in Alzheimer's Disease. *J Clin Endocrinol Metab.* 1997;82(10):3251-3259.

176. Squire LR, Stark CEL, Clark RE. The Medial Temporal Lobe. *Annual Review of Neuroscience.* 2004;27(1):279-306.

177. Bremner JD, Narayan M, Anderson ER, Staib LH, Miller HL, Charney DS. Hippocampal Volume Reduction in Major Depression. *Am J Psychiatry.* 2000;157(1):115-118.

178. Frenkel GD, Harrington L. Inhibition of mitochondrial nucleic acid synthesis by methyl mercury. *Biochem Pharmacol.* Apr 15 1983;32(8):1454-1456.

179. Yee S, Choi BH. Oxidative stress in neurotoxic effects of methylmercury poisoning. *Neurotoxicology.* Spring 1996;17(1):17-26.

180. Dimopoulos N, Piperi C, Salonicioti A, et al. Association of cognitive impairment with plasma levels of folate, vitamin B12 and homocysteine in the elderly. *In Vivo.* Nov-Dec 2006;20(6B):895-899.

181. Overweight and obesity. Web page]. June 25, 2004; http://www.cdc.gov/nccdphp/dnpa/obesity/. Accessed March 28, 2005.

182. Hedley AA, Ogden CL, Johnson CL, Carroll MD, Curtin LR, Flegal KM. Prevalence of Overweight and Obesity Among U.S. Children, Adolescents, and Adults, 1999-2002. *JAMA.* 2004;291(23):2847-2850.

183. Ogden CL, Carroll MD, Curtin LR, McDowell MA, Tabak CJ, Flegal KM. Prevalence of Overweight and Obesity in the United States, 1999-2004 10.1001/jama.295.13.1549. *JAMA.* 2006;295(13):1549-1555.

184. Wurtman RJ, Wurtman JJ. Brain serotonin, carbohydrate-craving, obesity and depression. *Obes Res.* Nov 1995;3 Suppl 4:477S-480S.

185. Laurant P, Touyz RM, Schiffrin EL. Effect of magnesium on vascular tone and reactivity in pressurized mesenteric resistance arteries from spontaneously hypertensive rats. *Can J Physiol Pharmacol.* Apr 1997;75(4):293-300.

186. Northcott CA, Watts SW. Low [Mg2+]e enhances arterial spontaneous tone via phosphatidylinositol 3-kinase in DOCA-salt hypertension. *Hypertension.* Jan 2004;43(1):125-129.

187. Touyz RM, Laurant P, Schiffrin EL. Effect of magnesium on calcium responses to vasopressin in vascular smooth muscle cells of spontaneously hypertensive rats. *J Pharmacol Exp Ther.* Mar 1998;284(3):998-1005.

188. Yang ZW, Wang J, Zheng T, Altura BT, Altura BM. Low [Mg(2+)](o) induces contraction and [Ca(2+)](i) rises in cerebral arteries: roles of ca(2+), PKC, and PI3. *Am J Physiol Heart Circ Physiol.* Dec 2000;279(6):H2898-2907.

189. Toda N, Ayajiki K, Okamura T. Nitric oxide and penile erectile function. *Pharmacol Ther.* May 2005;106(2):233-266.

190. Siroen MPC, Teerlink T, Nijveldt RJ, Prins HA, Richir MC, Leeuwen PAMv. The Clinical Significance of Asymmetric Dimethylarginine. *Ann Rev Nutr.* 2006;26(1):203-228.

191. Matz R. Hypoglycemia, seizures, and pulmonary edema. *Diabetes Care.* 2000;23(11):1715b-.

192. Kirchner A, Veliskova J, Velisek L. Differential effects of low glucose concentrations on seizures and epileptiform activity in vivo and in vitro. *Eur J Neurosci.* Mar 2006;23(6):1512-1522.

193. Monami M, Mannucci E, Breschi A, Marchionni N. Seizures as the only clinical manifestation of reactive hypoglycemia: a case report. *J Endocrinol Invest.* Nov 2005;28(10):940-941.

194. Tamura Y, Araki A, Chiba Y, Horiuchi T, Mori S, Hosoi T. Postprandial reactive hypoglycemia in an oldest-old patient effectively treated with low-dose acarbose. *Endocr J.* Dec 2006;53(6):767-771.

195. Brun JF, Fedou C, Mercier J. Postprandial reactive hypoglycemia. *Diabetes Metab.* Nov 2000;26(5):337-351.

196. Chan JM, Stampfer MJ, Ma J, Gann PH, Gaziano JM, Giovannucci EL. Dairy products, calcium, and prostate cancer risk in the Physicians' Health Study. *Am J Clin Nutr.* 2001;74(4):549-554.

197. Muti P, Bradlow HL, Micheli A, et al. Estrogen metabolism and risk of breast cancer: a prospective study of the 2:16alpha-hydroxyestrone ratio in premenopausal and postmenopausal women. *Epidemiology.* Nov 2000;11(6):635-640.

198. Dalessandri KM, Firestone GL, Fitch MD, Bradlow HL, Bjeldanes LF. Pilot Study: Effect of 3,3'-Diindolylmethane Supplements on Urinary Hormone Metabolites in Postmenopausal Women With a History of Early-Stage Breast Cancer. *Nutrition and Cancer.* 2004;50(2):161-167.

Index

978-0-595-45340-5
0-595-45340-6

Made in the USA
Las Vegas, NV
26 February 2021